I CAN BE A
HANDFULL

A CARER'S GUIDE TO MALE PERSONAL CARE

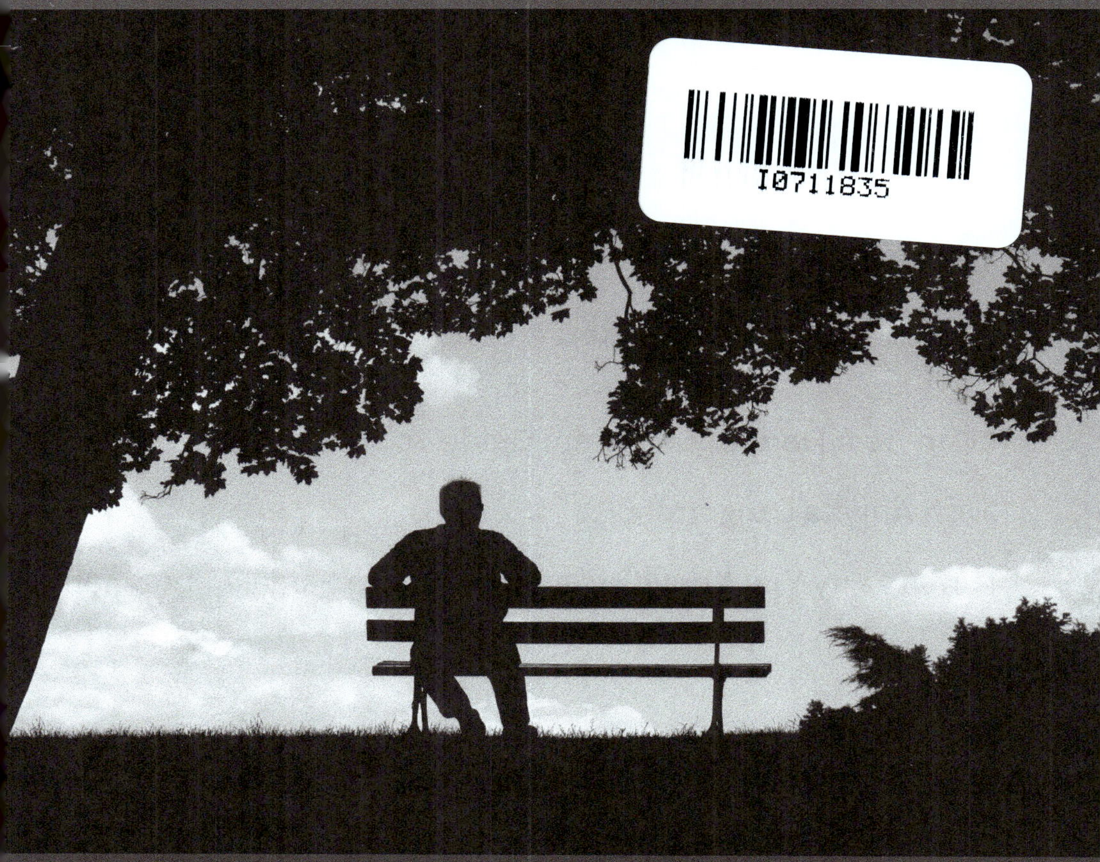

ROY LANGSTAFFE

I Can Be A Handful

A Carers Guide to Male Personal Care

Roy Langstaffe

I Can Be A Handful.

A CARER'S GUIDE TO MALE PERSONAL CARE:

Hello, I'm Roy Langstaffe, a seasoned trainer and coach with a deep passion for caregiving. With years of experience, I excel in guiding individuals to become exceptional caregivers.

I collaborate with diverse organizations to elevate caregiving standards and practices. Beyond my training endeavors, I'm also an author and aspiring musician, showcasing my multifaceted approach to life.

My commitment to the well-being of caregivers is evident in my tireless advocacy and dedication. With compassion and creativity at the forefront, I strive to make a meaningful impact on the lives of caregivers and those they care for, ensuring their sanity and strength are upheld.

I hope you enjoy this book and find some knowledge that helps you!

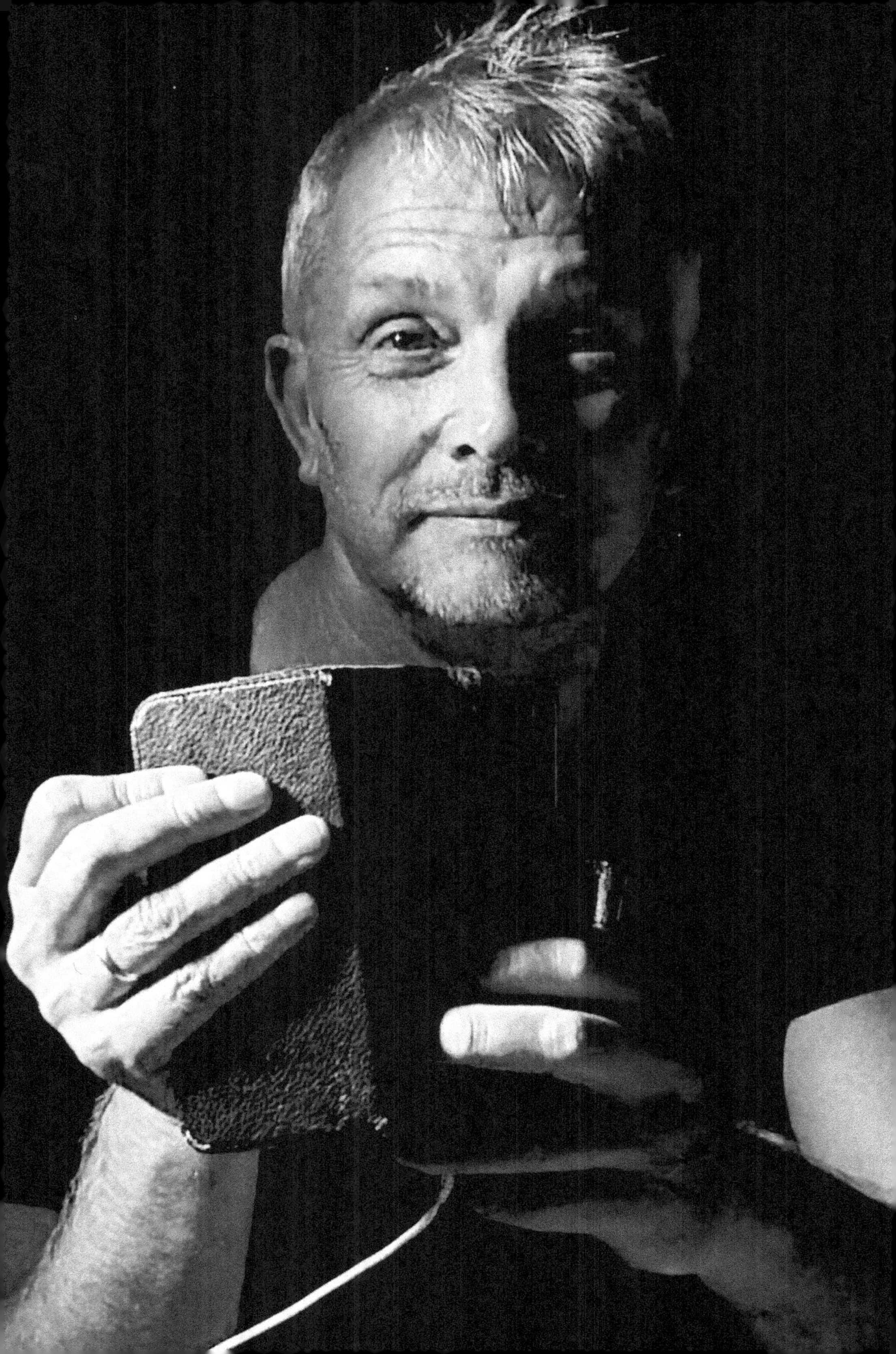

CHAPTER 1: INTRODUCTION

Understanding the Unique Needs of Male Care Recipients

In the timeless words of James Brown, "This is a man's world, but it wouldn't be nothing without a woman or a girl." While this anthem resonates with the societal landscape, it also sheds light on the complexities and challenges faced by men, particularly in the realm of personal care. In caregiving, understanding these nuances is crucial to providing effective support.

Men, like women, have distinct care requirements that stem from biological, social, and psychological factors. From navigating the impact of traditional masculine norms to addressing specific health concerns, male care recipients often encounter unique challenges. These challenges necessitate a thoughtful and tailored approach to caregiving that goes beyond the surface.

Overview of Male-Specific Care Challenges

Male-specific care encompasses a spectrum of needs ranging from physical health to emotional well-being. Issues such as prostate health, male-pattern baldness, and the emotional impact of aging can significantly influence their care journey. Understanding and addressing these challenges proactively can enhance the quality of care provided.

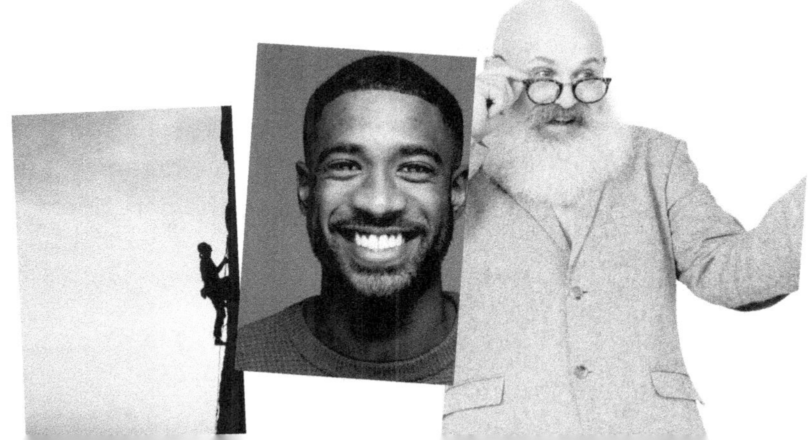

Importance of Tailored Approaches in Male Personal Care

Importance of Tailored Approaches in Male Personal Care
One size does not fit all when it comes to caregiving, especially for men. Tailoring care approaches to meet individual preferences, cultural backgrounds, and personal routines is essential for fostering trust and ensuring comfort. By acknowledging and accommodating these differences, caregivers can create environments that support men in maintaining their dignity and independence.

As we delve into the intricacies of male personal care, this guide aims to equip caregivers with the knowledge and insights needed to navigate these challenges with compassion and competence. Together, we can redefine caregiving as a collaborative journey that honours and meets the unique needs of every individual.

The Hang-ups Men Can Have When Being Cared For

Men often face unique emotional and psychological challenges when receiving care, rooted in societal expectations and personal beliefs about masculinity and independence. These hang-ups can manifest in various ways, creating obstacles in the caregiving relationship. In this guide, we will explore these issues in depth, providing insights and strategies to help caregivers navigate these complexities effectively.

Reluctance to Show Vulnerability: Many men are conditioned to equate vulnerability with weakness, leading to resistance when they need help with personal tasks such as bathing, dressing, or managing incontinence. This reluctance can hinder effective caregiving and create tension between the care recipient and the caregiver.

Concerns About Loss of Independence: The fear of losing independence is a significant concern for many men. Being dependent on someone else for daily activities can lead to feelings of frustration, helplessness, and even depression. Understanding and addressing these fears is crucial for providing compassionate care.

Privacy and Dignity Issues: Maintaining privacy and dignity is essential for all care recipients, but it can be particularly challenging for men who may feel embarrassed or uncomfortable with intimate care tasks. This can be exacerbated when the caregiver is a family member, adding a layer of complexity to the caregiving dynamic.

Difficulty Expressing Emotions: Men may struggle to express their emotions or articulate their needs due to societal norms that discourage emotional openness. This can lead to misunderstandings and unmet needs, impacting the quality of care they receive.

Challenges for Carers:

Caring for a male family member, such as a father or brother, comes with its own set of challenges. Caregivers may face emotional strain, boundary issues, and role reversal difficulties. Balancing respect for the care recipient's independence with the need to provide necessary support can be particularly challenging.

Emotional Strain and Role Reversal: Caring for a father, brother, or another male relative can be emotionally taxing, especially when dealing with the role reversal of becoming a caregiver for someone who once cared for you. This shift can lead to feelings of guilt, sadness, and frustration.

Boundary Issues: Maintaining appropriate boundaries while providing intimate care can be difficult, especially for female caregivers. Ensuring the comfort and dignity of both the caregiver and the care recipient is essential, yet challenging.

Conclusion

In the coming chapters, we will delve deeper into these hang-ups and challenges, providing practical advice and strategies to help caregivers manage these situations with empathy and effectiveness. From establishing trust and open communication to navigating the intricacies of personal care tasks, this guide will equip you with the tools needed to provide the best possible care for the men in your life.

So, as we continue our journey through "I can Be A Handful", we will explore a number of areas that you need to be aware of, including personal hygiene and care, and the essentail things you need to know on how to support someone.

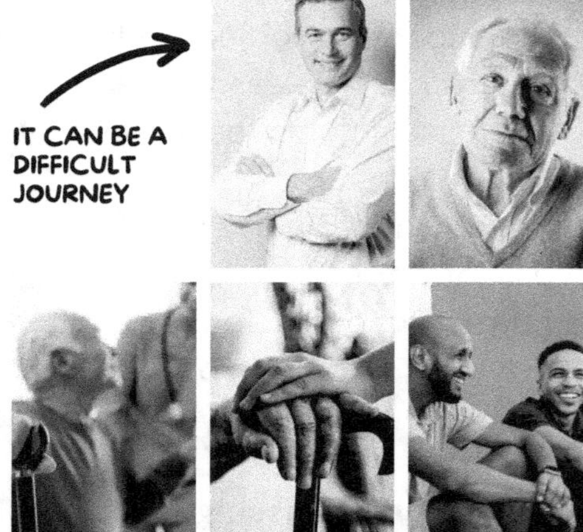

BUT THEY NEED YOU!

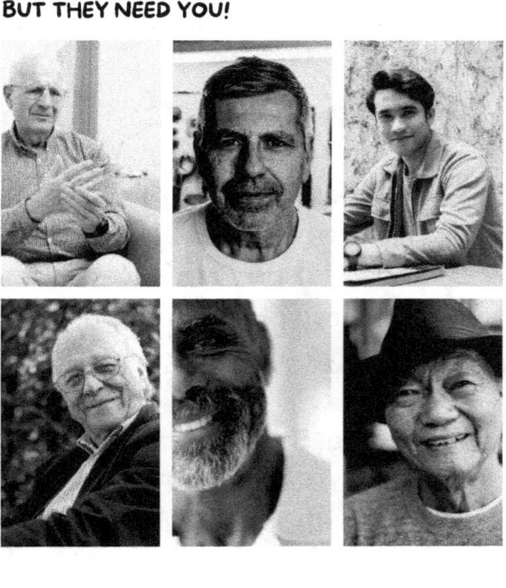

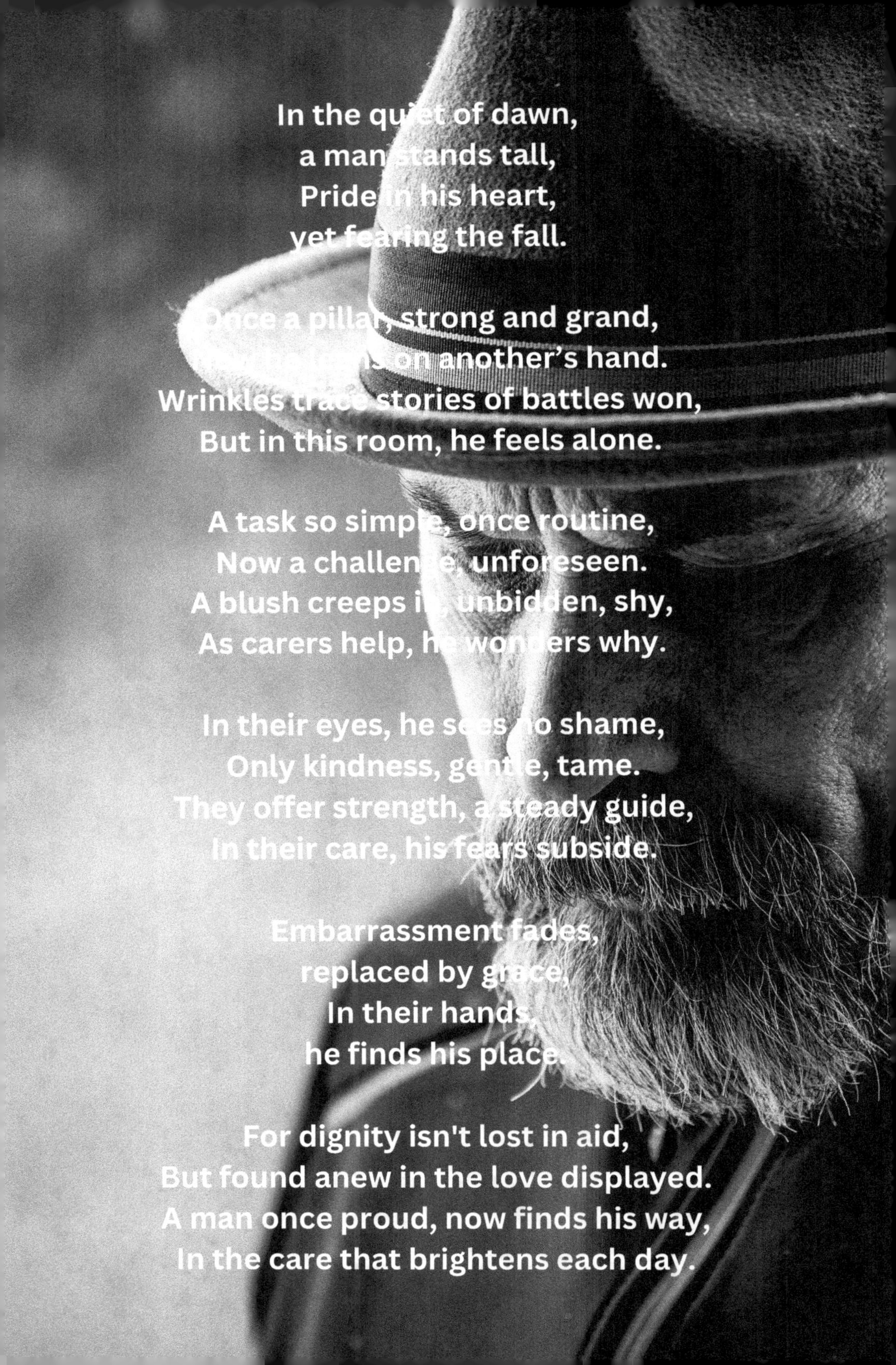

In the quiet of dawn,
a man stands tall,
Pride in his heart,
yet fearing the fall.

Once a pillar, strong and grand,
Now he leans on another's hand.
Wrinkles trace stories of battles won,
But in this room, he feels alone.

A task so simple, once routine,
Now a challenge, unforeseen.
A blush creeps in, unbidden, shy,
As carers help, he wonders why.

In their eyes, he sees no shame,
Only kindness, gentle, tame.
They offer strength, a steady guide,
In their care, his fears subside.

Embarrassment fades,
replaced by grace,
In their hands,
he finds his place.

For dignity isn't lost in aid,
But found anew in the love displayed.
A man once proud, now finds his way,
In the care that brightens each day.

CHAPTER 2: ESTABLISHING TRUST AND COMMUNICATION

Building Rapport with Male Care Recipients

Building rapport with male care recipients can differ significantly from establishing connections with female care recipients. Men often have unique experiences, emotions, and worldviews shaped by societal expectations and personal history. Understanding these differences is crucial for creating a trusting and effective caregiving relationship.

For many older men, traditional roles meant that they went to work and were often separate from family life. This separation can influence how they interact with caregivers, particularly if they are not used to sharing personal or emotional aspects of their lives. Establishing rapport, therefore, requires sensitivity to these generational and cultural contexts.

Start with Shared Interests: Engage in conversations about topics they enjoy or are passionate about, such as hobbies, sports, or past careers. Finding common ground can help break the ice and build a foundation of mutual respect and understanding.

Be Patient and Consistent: Trust takes time to develop, especially if the care recipient is initially resistant. Demonstrating reliability and consistency in your actions and communication helps to build trust gradually.

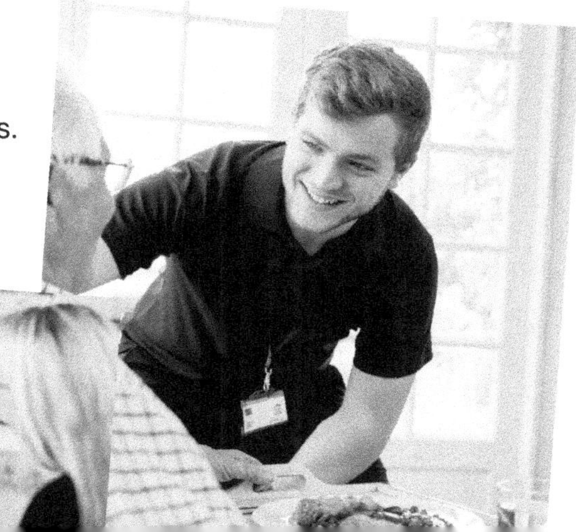

Show Respect for Their Experiences: Acknowledge and respect their life experiences and achievements. This validation can help them feel valued and understood. Everyone experience things from a different perspective, so it is important that you try to see things from their point of view.

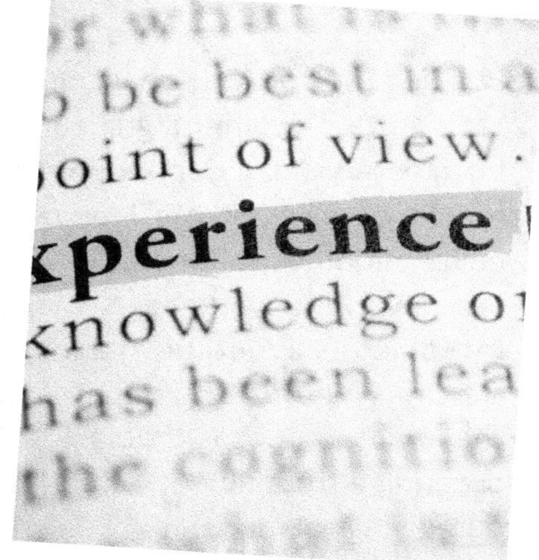

Overcoming Communication Barriers

Communication barriers can arise from a variety of sources, including generational differences, personal discomfort with expressing emotions, or cognitive impairments. Overcoming these barriers is essential for effective caregiving.

Use Clear and Simple Language: Avoid jargon and complex sentences. Speak clearly and directly to ensure that your message is understood. This can be easier with relatives who share a common background, but as a carer looking after a non-relative, especially someone from another part of the country, this can be more difficult. They may have a strong accent or use different words. For example, in England, the evening meal is known as "dinner" in the south, while in parts of the north, it can be called "tea" or "supper."

Be Attentive to Non-Verbal Cues: Men might express discomfort or needs through body language rather than words. Pay attention to these cues and respond accordingly.

Encourage Open Dialogue: Create an environment where the care recipient feels safe to express their thoughts and feelings. Encourage them to share their preferences and concerns without fear of judgment.

Adapt to Their Communication Style: Some men may prefer brief, straightforward conversations, while others might open up more with time. Tailor your communication style to their preferences.

Incorporate Interests and Common Ground: Men can often have different interests, such as football (soccer) and other sports. Engaging in conversations about these interests can help bridge communication gaps. Building in interests and finding common ground can make the care recipient feel more comfortable and understood, thereby easing communication barriers.

Respecting Privacy and Dignity

Respecting a care recipient's privacy and dignity is fundamental to maintaining their self-esteem and comfort. This is particularly important when providing intimate care or discussing personal matters. This can also include knocking before entering their personal space and announce your intentions. This shows respect for their privacy.

Explain What You're Doing: Before performing any care tasks, explain what you will be doing and why. This helps the care recipient feel more in control and less anxious about the process. Recognize and respect their comfort levels with physical contact and personal care tasks. If they seem uncomfortable, ask for their preferences and adjust your approach accordingly.

Provide Options and Choices: Whenever possible, offer choices about how and when care is provided. This can help the care recipient feel more autonomous and respected.

Conclusion

In summary, establishing trust and effective communication with male care recipients involves understanding their unique backgrounds and experiences, overcoming communication barriers with patience and adaptability, and consistently respecting their privacy and dignity.

By focusing on these aspects, caregivers can foster a positive and supportive environment that enhances the quality of care provided. Remeber to put yourself in their shoes. The only person who may have ever seen them naked is their wife. All of a sudden they are having to expose themselves to a stranger or a daughter or son, and reveal details about bowel movements or how they feel.

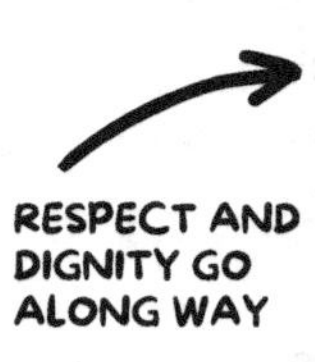

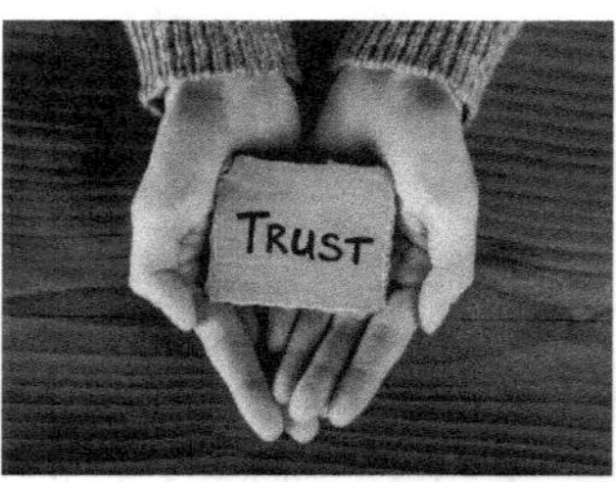

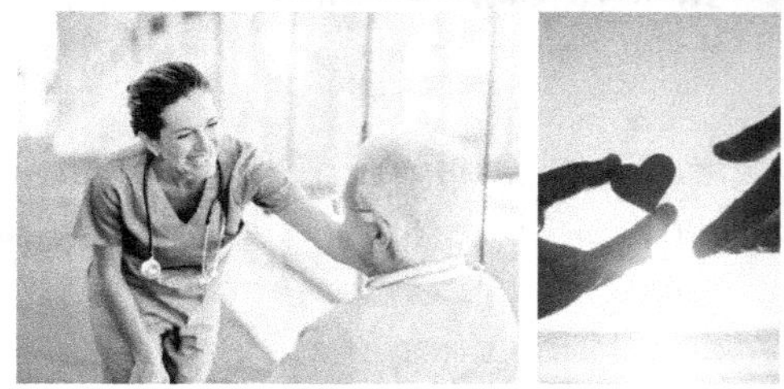

MSEE THE PERSON, NOT THE CONDITION

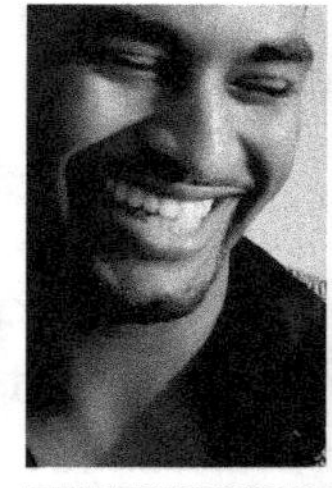

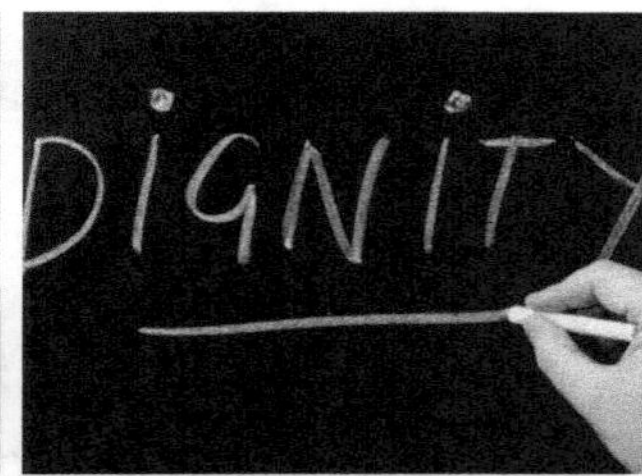

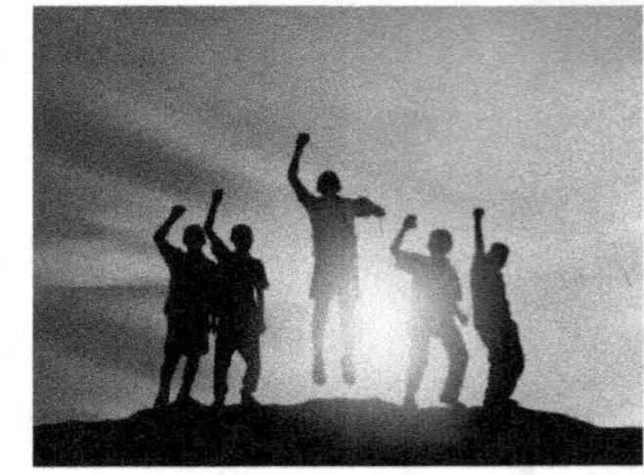

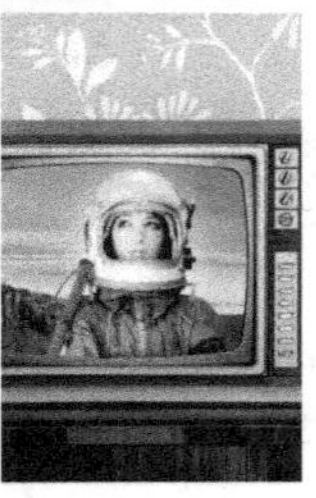

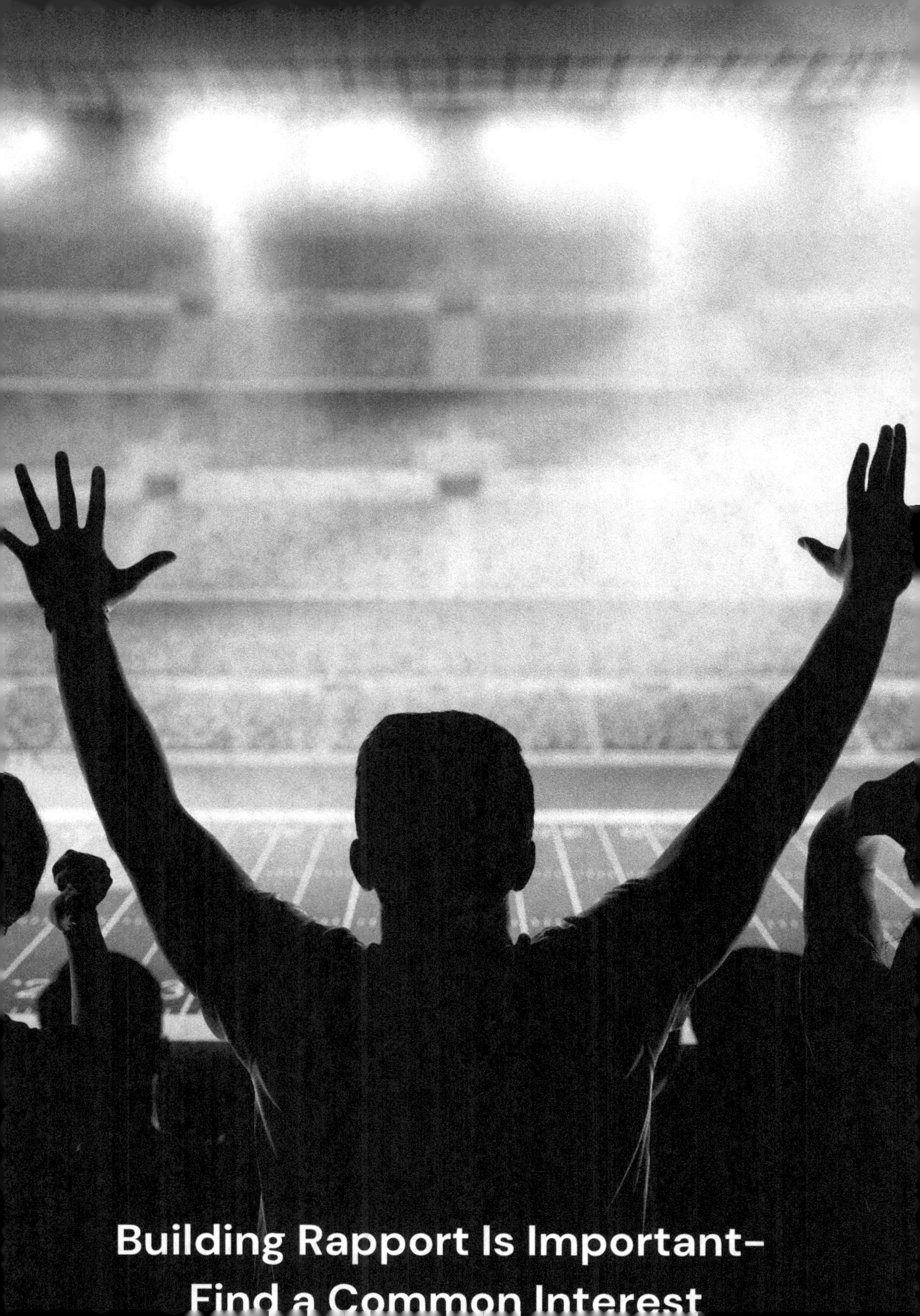
Building Rapport Is Important–
Find a Common Interest

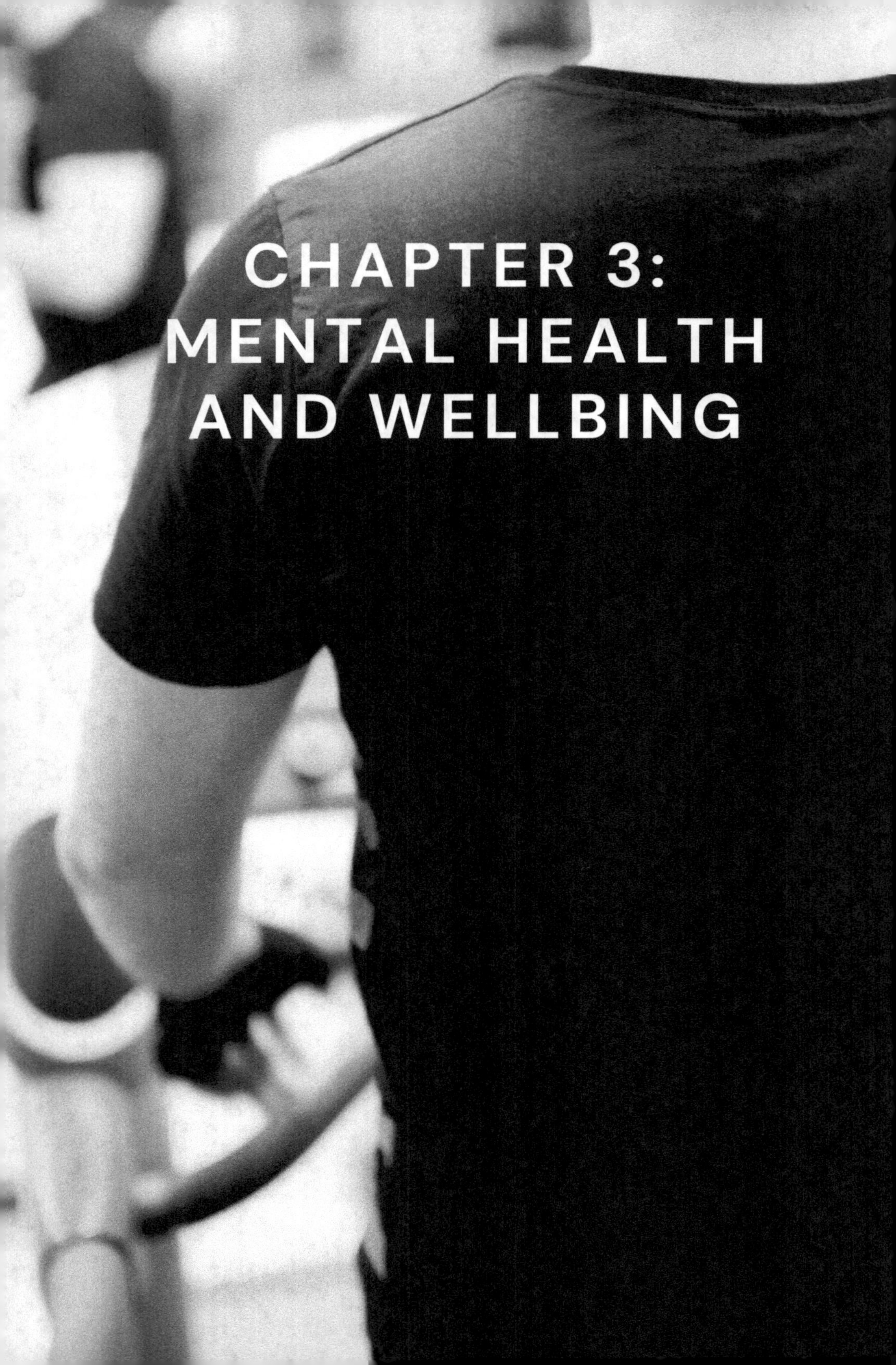
CHAPTER 3:
MENTAL HEALTH
AND WELLBING

Recognizing Signs of Depression and Anxiety in Men

Men, particularly from older generations, often find it challenging to talk about their concerns and emotional struggles. They were frequently encouraged to suppress their feelings and "tough it out." As a result, many men may not openly express signs of depression or anxiety, making it crucial for caregivers to recognize these signs through observation and subtle cues.

Changes in Mood and Behaviour: Look for signs such as persistent sadness, irritability, or anger. Men might also withdraw from social activities they previously enjoyed or exhibit a lack of interest in daily life.

Physical Symptoms: Depression and anxiety in men can manifest as physical symptoms, including unexplained aches and pains, changes in appetite or sleep patterns, and fatigue.

Expression of Hopelessness: Pay attention to statements that reflect a sense of hopelessness or worthlessness. These can be direct comments or more subtle hints about feeling like a burden or questioning their purpose.

Increased Substance Use: Some men may turn to alcohol or other substances to cope with their feelings. An increase in substance use can be a red flag for underlying mental health issues.

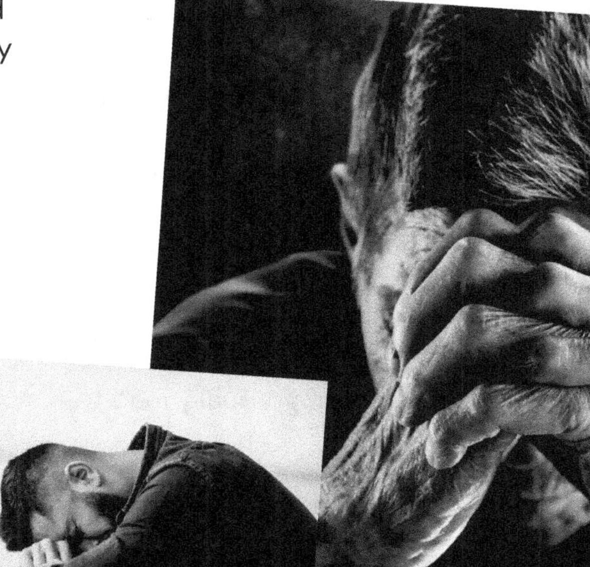

Understanding the reasons why men may not communicate their feelings is crucial. Generally, they fall into three categories:

They Won't: They choose not to share their problems, often due to pride or societal conditioning.

They Can't: They are unable to communicate due to a condition or communication barriers.

They Will: They are willing to open up, often as a result of established trust.

Supporting Mental Health Through Active Listening and Empathy

Understanding the psychological impact of losing independence and feeling misunderstood is vital in supporting a man's mental health. Imagine being independent your whole life and suddenly needing care, or feeling like no one understands you. These experiences can significantly affect mental wellbeing.

Active Listening: Show genuine interest in their thoughts and feelings. Practice active listening by giving them your full attention, nodding, and providing verbal affirmations without interrupting. This helps them feel heard and valued.

Empathy and Understanding: Acknowledge their feelings and validate their experiences. Empathy involves understanding their perspective and showing compassion for their struggles.

Encouraging Expression: Create a safe space for them to express their concerns and emotions. Encourage them to talk about their day, their memories, or any worries they might have.

Establishing trust is essential in helping men feel comfortable enough to share their concerns. Building rapport and demonstrating reliability can gradually lead to a more open dialogue.

Encouraging Social Interaction and Engagement

Social isolation can exacerbate feelings of depression and anxiety. Encouraging social interaction and engagement can significantly improve mental health and wellbeing.

Facilitate Social Activities: Encourage participation in social activities that interest them, such as joining a local club, attending community events, or engaging in hobbies with others.

Connect with Family and Friends: Help maintain and strengthen connections with family and friends. Regular visits, phone calls, or video chats can provide emotional support and reduce feelings of loneliness.

Group Activities: Consider organizing group activities, like exercise classes, book clubs, or discussion groups, where they can interact with others in a relaxed setting.

Accessing Professional Mental Health Resources

While caregivers play a crucial role in supporting mental health, professional help is often necessary for more severe cases of depression and anxiety.

Consulting a Healthcare Professional: Encourage the care recipient to speak with a healthcare professional about their mental health. A doctor can provide a diagnosis and recommend appropriate treatment options. Professional therapy or counselling can be very beneficial. Therapists can offer strategies to cope with depression and anxiety and provide a safe space for men to talk about their feelings.

Support Groups: Consider suggesting support groups specifically for men, where they can share their experiences and learn from others facing similar challenges.

Medication: In some cases, medication may be necessary to manage symptoms of depression and anxiety. A healthcare professional can assess the need for medication and monitor its effectiveness.

Conclusion

In summary, supporting the mental health and wellbeing of male care recipients requires recognizing the subtle signs of depression and anxiety, offering active listening and empathy, encouraging social interaction, and accessing professional mental health resources. By addressing these aspects and understanding the different ways men might or might not communicate their struggles, caregivers can help men navigate the emotional challenges of being cared for, ensuring they feel understood, respected, and valued.

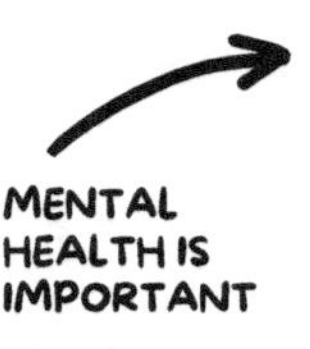

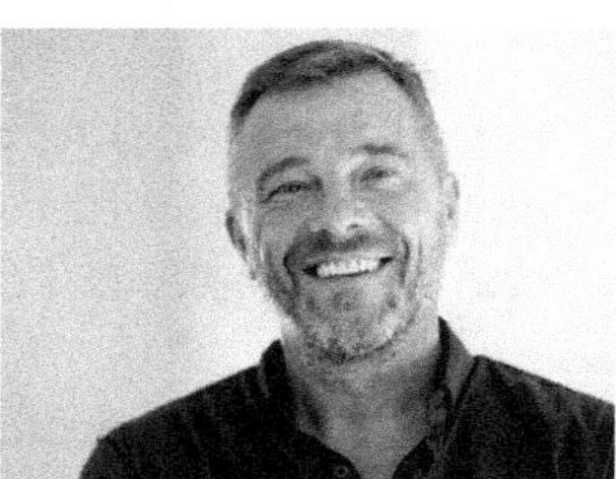

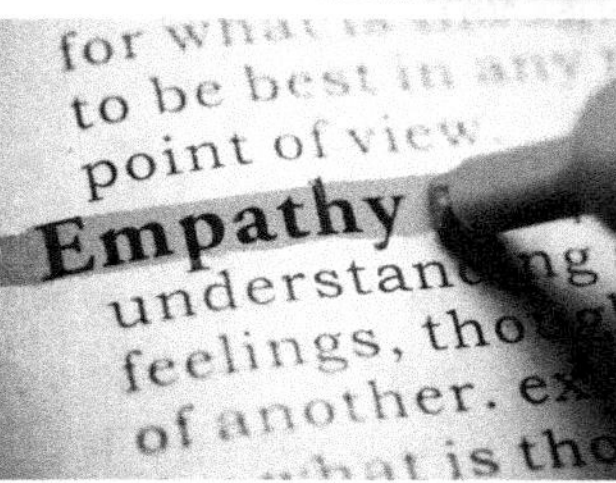

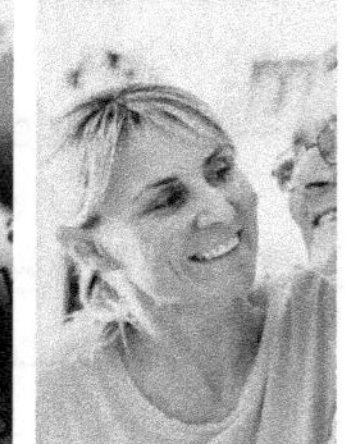

UNDERSTANDING MEN

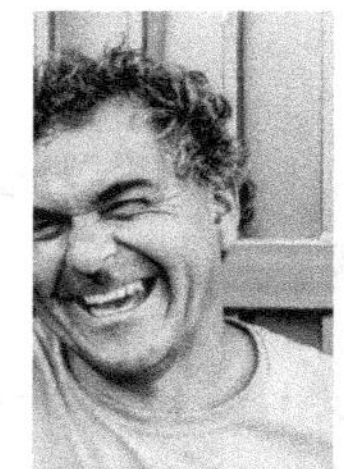

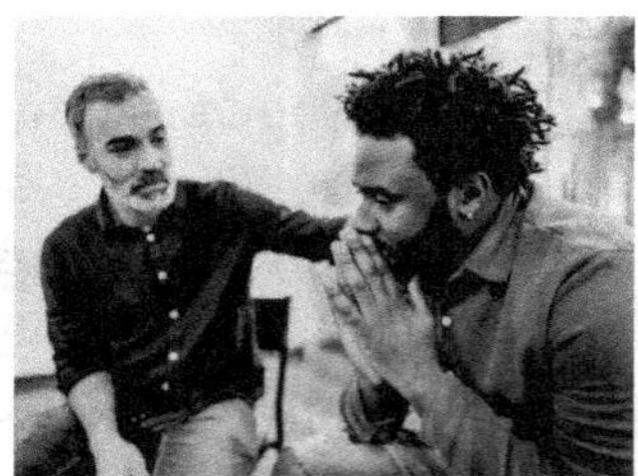

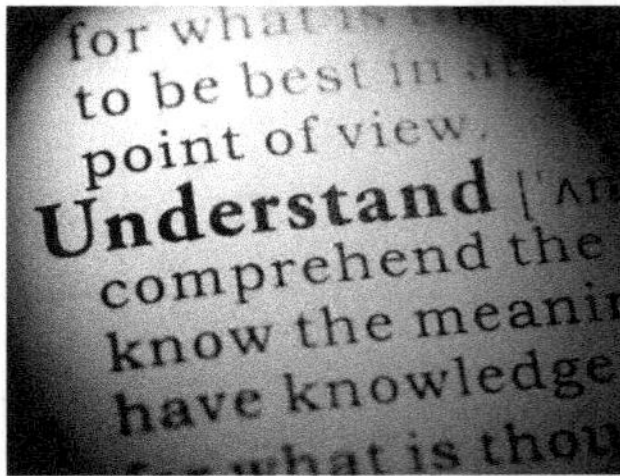

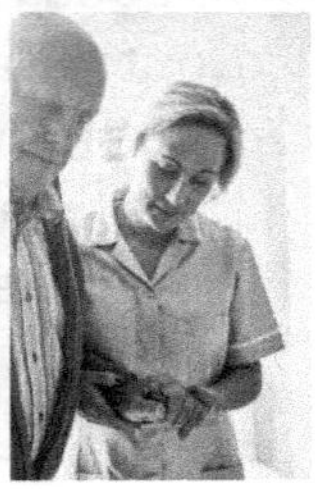

"As carers, we nurture not just the body, but the spirit. Supporting men's wellbeing means honoring their journey, embracing their vulnerability, and empowering their strength through compassion and understanding."

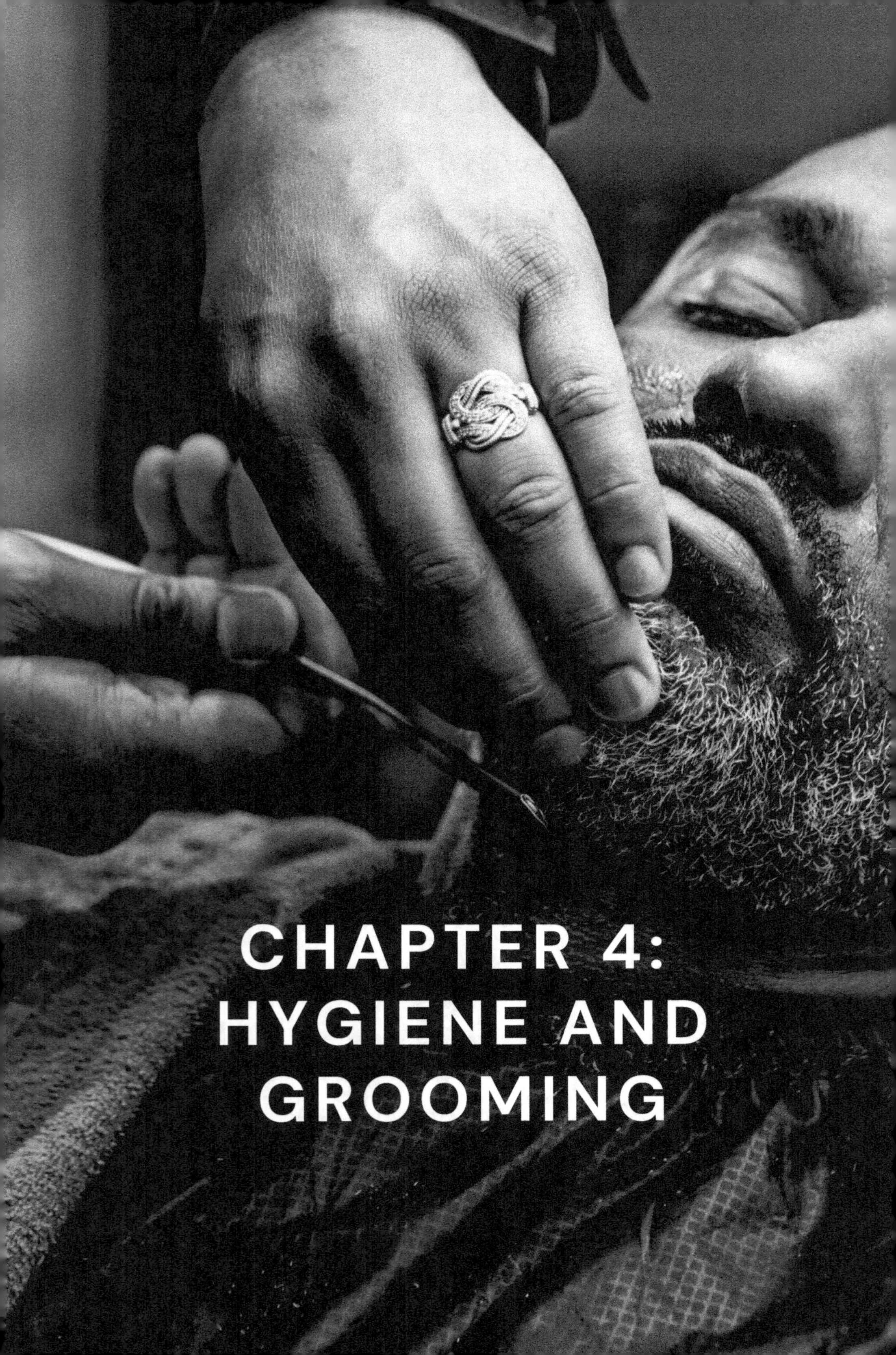

CHAPTER 4:
HYGIENE AND GROOMING

Daily Hygiene Routines: Bathing, Shaving, and Skincare

Maintaining good hygiene and grooming is essential for everyone, but it holds particular significance for men who may be adjusting to receiving care. Ensuring that male care recipients feel good about themselves through proper hygiene and grooming can boost their self-esteem, improve their mental health, and enhance their overall quality of life.

Daily Hygiene Routines: Bathing, Shaving, and Skincare

Establishing and maintaining daily hygiene routines is a fundamental aspect of personal care. These routines help in promoting physical health and psychological well-being. Here's a detailed guide on assisting someone with these routines while promoting as much independence as possible.

Independence

People go through life learning to be independent. People learn to talk, learn to eat, learn to dress, wash themselves and they make their own choices.

Imagine that being take away from you. Image that loss of independence. If you stop using your life skills, then people start to lose their indepedence and become reliant on you.

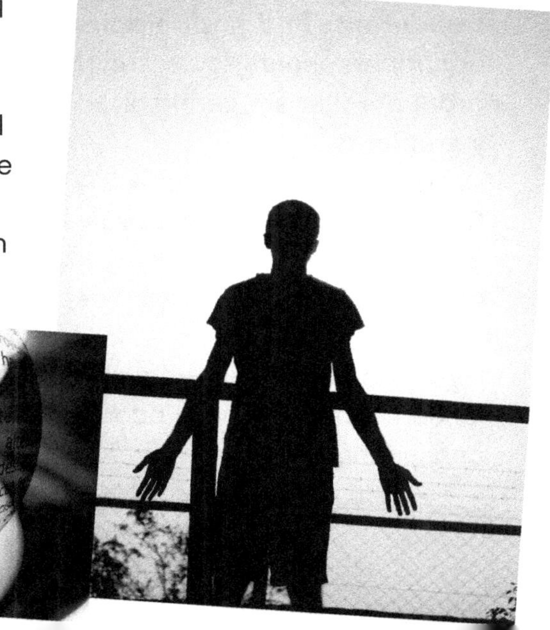

Managing Body Odour and Perspiration

Body odour and excessive perspiration can affect a man's self-confidence and social interactions. Managing these issues effectively is key to maintaining a positive self-image. Giving men a choice of toiletries and smells is important, as this will encourgage them to ensure this does not become a problem

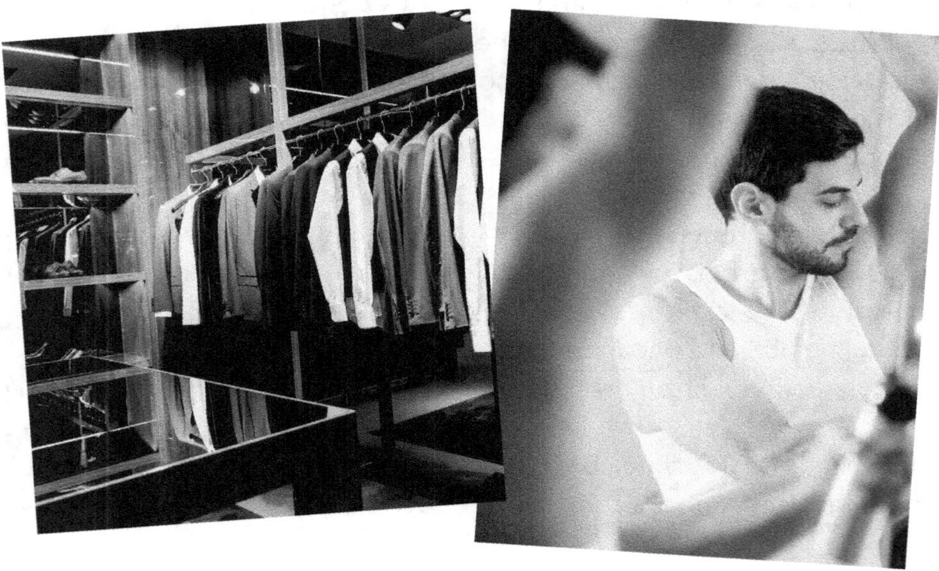

Deodorants and Antiperspirants: Encourage the use of deodorants or antiperspirants to control body odour and perspiration. Choose products that are gentle on the skin and free from irritating ingredients.

Regular Clothing Changes: Ensure that clothing is changed regularly, especially after physical activity. Fresh, clean clothes help in managing body odour and keeping the skin healthy.

Hydration and Diet: Proper hydration and a balanced diet can influence body odour. Encourage drinking plenty of water and consuming a diet rich in fruits, vegetables, and lean proteins.

Bathing Tips

Preparation: Ensure the bathroom is safe and comfortable. Use non-slip mats, install grab bars, and have a shower chair or bench available if needed. Gather all necessary supplies (soap, washcloth, towels, and clean clothes) beforehand.

Assistance Level: Encourage the individual to do as much as they can independently. Offer assistance with tasks they find difficult.

Independent Bathing: If the person can bathe themselves, ensure they have everything within reach. Provide guidance and support as needed, but allow them to maintain control.

Partial Assistance: For those needing some help, assist with washing hard-to-reach areas while encouraging them to wash areas they can reach. Use a handheld showerhead for better control.

Full Assistance: For those who need full support, maintain their dignity by explaining each step and keeping them covered with a towel when possible. Be gentle and thorough, ensuring all areas are cleaned properly.

Post-Bathing: Help the individual dry off completely to prevent skin issues. Apply lotion to keep the skin moisturized and assist them in getting dressed if needed.

Shaving Tips

Preparation: Gather all necessary shaving supplies (razor, shaving cream, mirror, towel, and aftershave). Ensure good lighting and a comfortable, seated position.

Assistance Level: Encourage the individual to shave themselves if possible, providing assistance as needed.

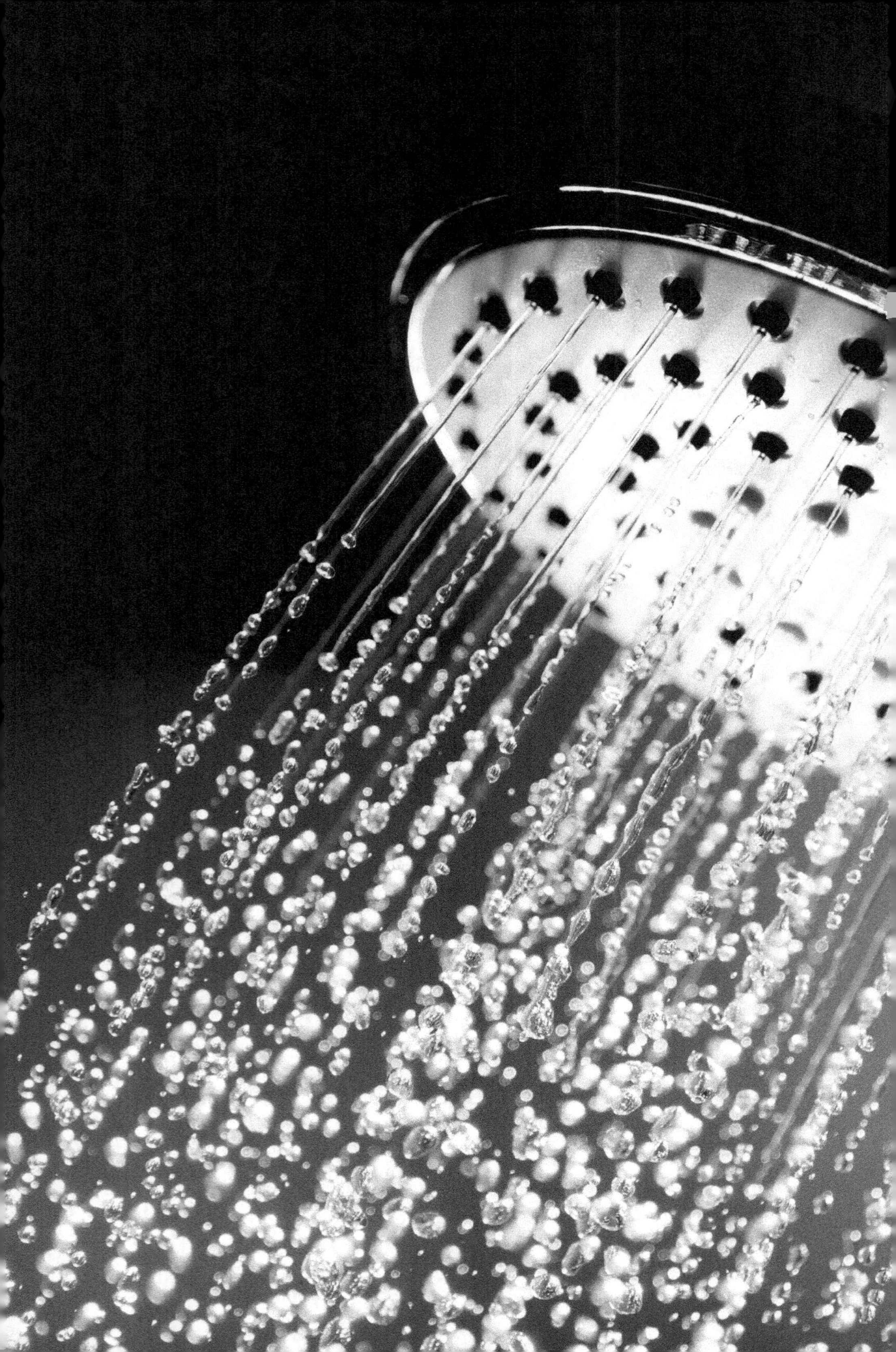

Independent Shaving: If the person can shave independently, ensure they have all supplies within reach and provide guidance on technique if necessary.

Partial Assistance: For those needing some help, assist with applying shaving cream and guide their hand if needed. Offer to shave difficult areas like under the chin or around the neck.

Full Assistance: For those who need full support, gently apply shaving cream and use a steady hand to shave. Use an electric razor for safety if the individual has unsteady hands or sensitive skin.

Post-Shaving: Rinse the face with warm water and apply aftershave or moisturizer to soothe the skin.

Skincare Tips

Daily Routine: Establish a simple daily skincare routine that includes cleansing, moisturizing, and sun protection.

Cleansing: Use a gentle cleanser suitable for the individual's skin type. Assist them in washing their face, paying special attention to areas prone to oiliness or dryness.

Moisturizing: Apply a moisturizer to keep the skin hydrated. Choose products that are appropriate for their skin type and any specific skin conditions they might have.

Sun Protection: Encourage the use of sunscreen with at least SPF 30 when going outdoors to protect the skin from harmful UV rays.

Weekly Routine: Incorporate exfoliation once or twice a week to remove dead skin cells and promote healthy skin regeneration. Use a mild exfoliator and assist as needed.

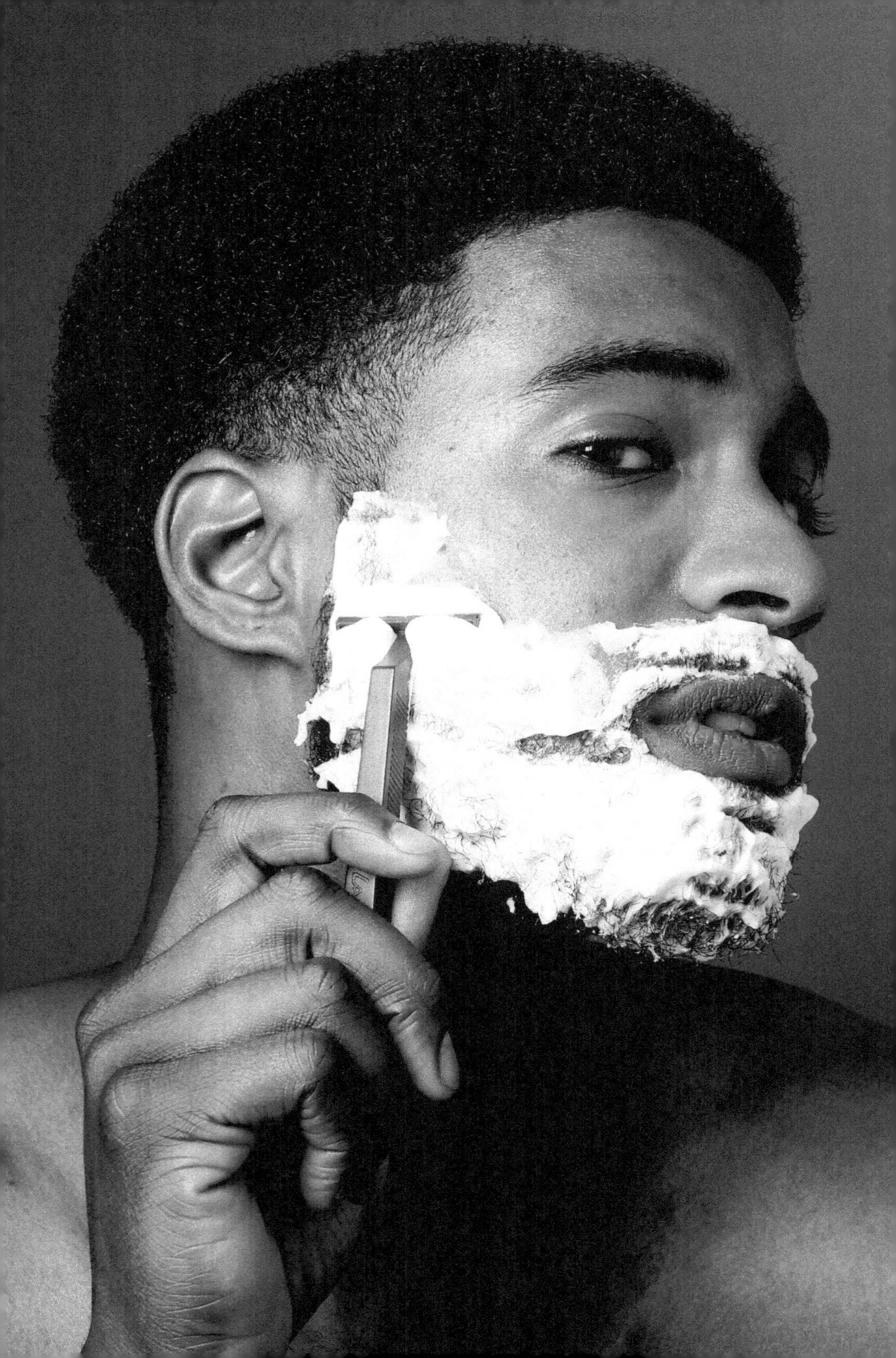

Hair Care: Washing, Cutting, and Styling

Hair care is an integral part of grooming and can significantly impact how a man feels about his appearance.

Washing: Regular hair washing helps keep the scalp clean and prevents dandruff. Use a mild shampoo suited to the individual's hair type and condition. For those who cannot wash their hair frequently, dry shampoo can be a useful alternative.

Assistance Level: Encourage the individual to wash their hair independently if possible. Provide support by handing them shampoo and offering to help rinse.

Full Assistance: If full assistance is needed, use a handheld showerhead for better control and ensure the water temperature is comfortable. Be gentle when massaging the scalp and thorough when rinsing.

Cutting: Regular haircuts help maintain a neat and tidy appearance. Whether the individual prefers short or long hair, keeping it trimmed prevents it from becoming unmanageable. Arrange for professional haircuts if possible, or learn basic haircutting techniques to assist them at home.

Professional Services: Schedule regular appointments with a barber or hairdresser.

Home Haircuts: If cutting hair at home, ensure you have the right tools and understand basic techniques. Offer regular trims to keep hair looking neat.

Styling: Styling can boost a man's confidence and sense of self. Help them style their hair according to their preferences using suitable products like gels, pomades, or hairsprays. Respect their personal style choices to ensure they feel good about their appearance.

Nail Care: Maintaining Clean and Trimmed Nails

Well-maintained nails are an important aspect of hygiene and grooming that is often overlooked. Clean and trimmed nails prevent infections and improve overall appearance.

Trimming: Regular nail trimming helps prevent nails from becoming too long and breaking or causing discomfort. Use clean, sharp nail clippers and file the edges to smooth out any roughness.

Assistance Level: Encourage the individual to trim their nails independently if possible. Offer guidance on technique and provide assistance with hard-to-reach toenails.

Full Assistance: For those who need full support, gently trim the nails, ensuring not to cut too short. File the edges to avoid sharp points.

Cleaning: Encourage regular cleaning of nails to remove dirt and prevent bacterial or fungal infections. Use a soft nail brush and mild soap to clean under the nails.

Daily Care: Incorporate nail cleaning into the daily hygiene routine.

Weekly Care: Perform a thorough cleaning and trimming once a week to maintain nail health.

Hand and Foot Care: Pay attention to both fingernails and toenails. For toenails, ensure they are cut straight across to prevent ingrown nails. Moisturize hands and feet to keep the skin soft and prevent dryness.

Moisturizing: Apply hand and foot cream regularly to maintain skin health.

Inspecting: Regularly inspect the nails and surrounding skin for any signs of infection or issues.

Conclusion

In conclusion, maintaining proper hygiene and grooming routines is essential for men to feel good about themselves.

Daily practices like bathing, shaving, and skincare, along with managing body odour, hair care, and nail care, contribute to their overall well-being.

By supporting male care recipients in these areas, caregivers can help them maintain their dignity, self-esteem, and quality of life while promoting as much independence as possible.

MAINTAINING PERSONAL HYGIENE

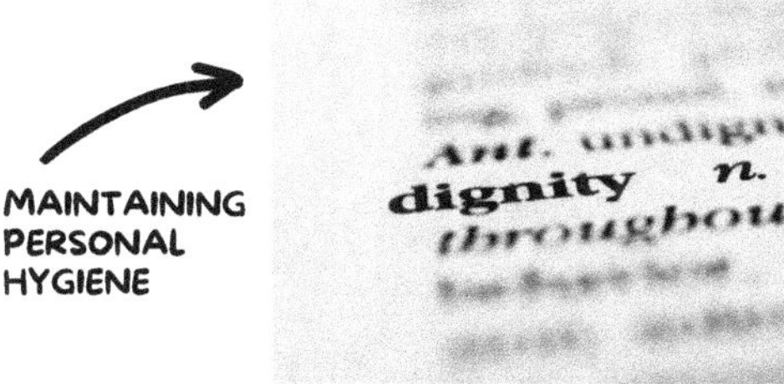

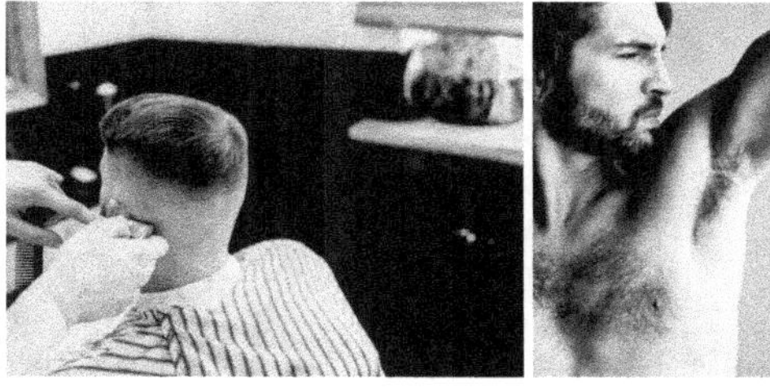

BRINGS DIGNITY AND EMPOWERMENT

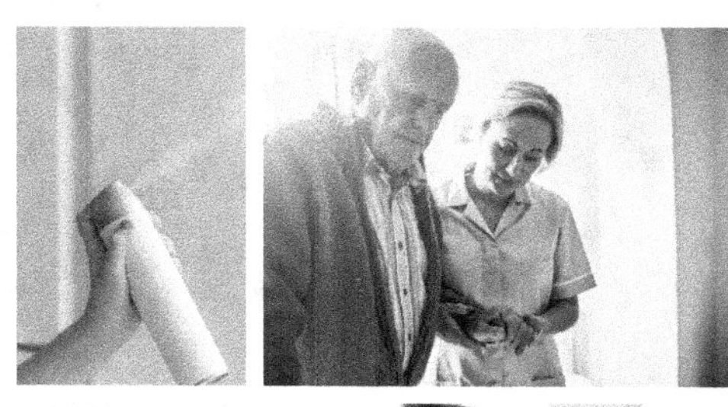

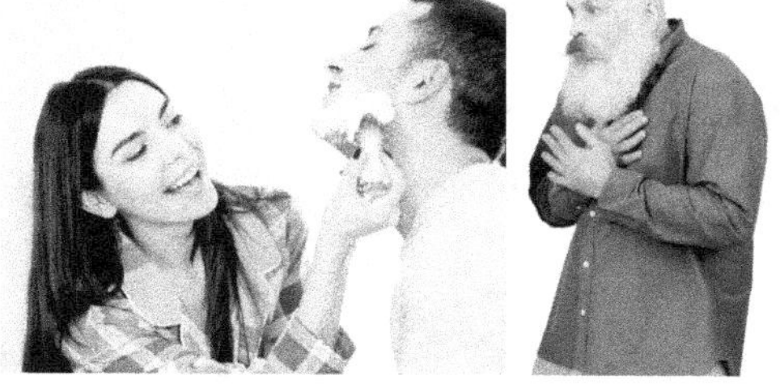

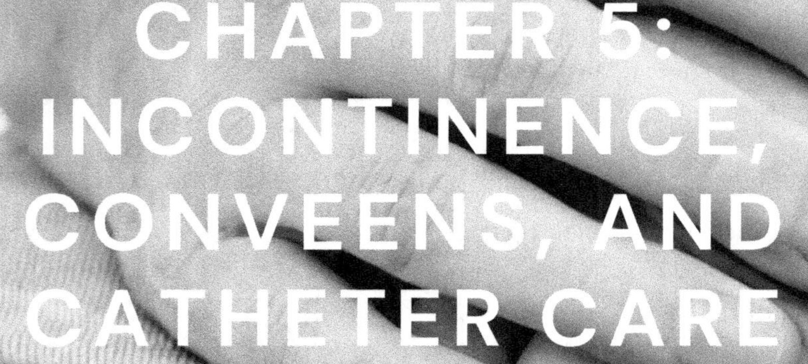

CHAPTER 5: INCONTINENCE, CONVEENS, AND CATHETER CARE

Understanding Urinary Incontinence in Men

Incontinence and catheter care can be significant sources of embarrassment and discomfort for men. It's crucial to approach these topics with sensitivity and use the correct terminology, such as "pads" instead of "nappies" or "diapers." Understanding these aspects and providing appropriate care can help maintain dignity and improve the quality of life for male care recipients.

Urinary incontinence is the involuntary leakage of urine, and it can affect men for various reasons, including age, prostate issues, or neurological conditions. Understanding the types and causes of incontinence is the first step in providing effective care.

Causes of Urinary Incontinence:

Prostate Problems: Enlarged prostate or prostate surgery can impact urinary control.

Neurological Disorders: Conditions such as Parkinson's disease, multiple sclerosis, or stroke can affect nerve signals involved in bladder control.

Medications: Certain medications can contribute to incontinence.

Types of Urinary Incontinence:

Stress Incontinence: Leakage occurs during activities that increase abdominal pressure, such as coughing, sneezing, or lifting heavy objects.

Urge Incontinence: A sudden, intense urge to urinate followed by involuntary leakage. This can be caused by overactive bladder muscles.

Overflow Incontinence: Inability to empty the bladder completely, leading to frequent dribbling of urine.

Functional Incontinence: Physical or mental impairment prevents timely access to a bathroom.

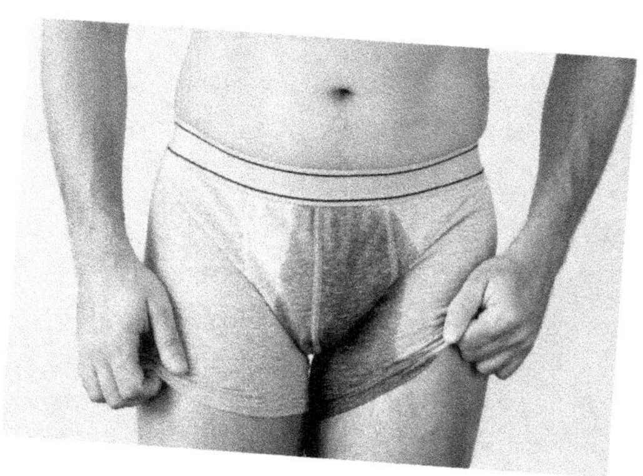

Types of Catheters and Their Appropriate Use

Catheters are medical devices used to drain urine from the bladder when an individual cannot do so naturally. These have been around for thousands of years and some of the earliest records date back to around 3000 BC during the Egyptian era.

Understanding the different types of catheters and their appropriate use is essential for effective care.

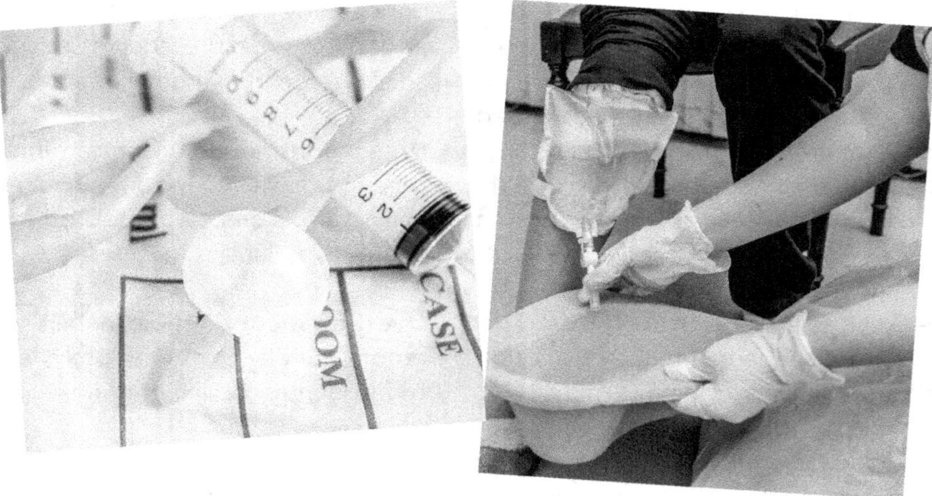

Intermittent Catheters: Used temporarily to drain the bladder and then removed. These are typically used for individuals who need to empty their bladder several times a day.

Indwelling Catheters (Foley Catheters): These are left in place for extended periods and held in the bladder by a small balloon. They are commonly used for individuals who cannot empty their bladder on their own.

Suprapubic Catheters: Inserted through a small incision in the abdomen directly into the bladder. These are used for long-term catheterization when other methods are not suitable.

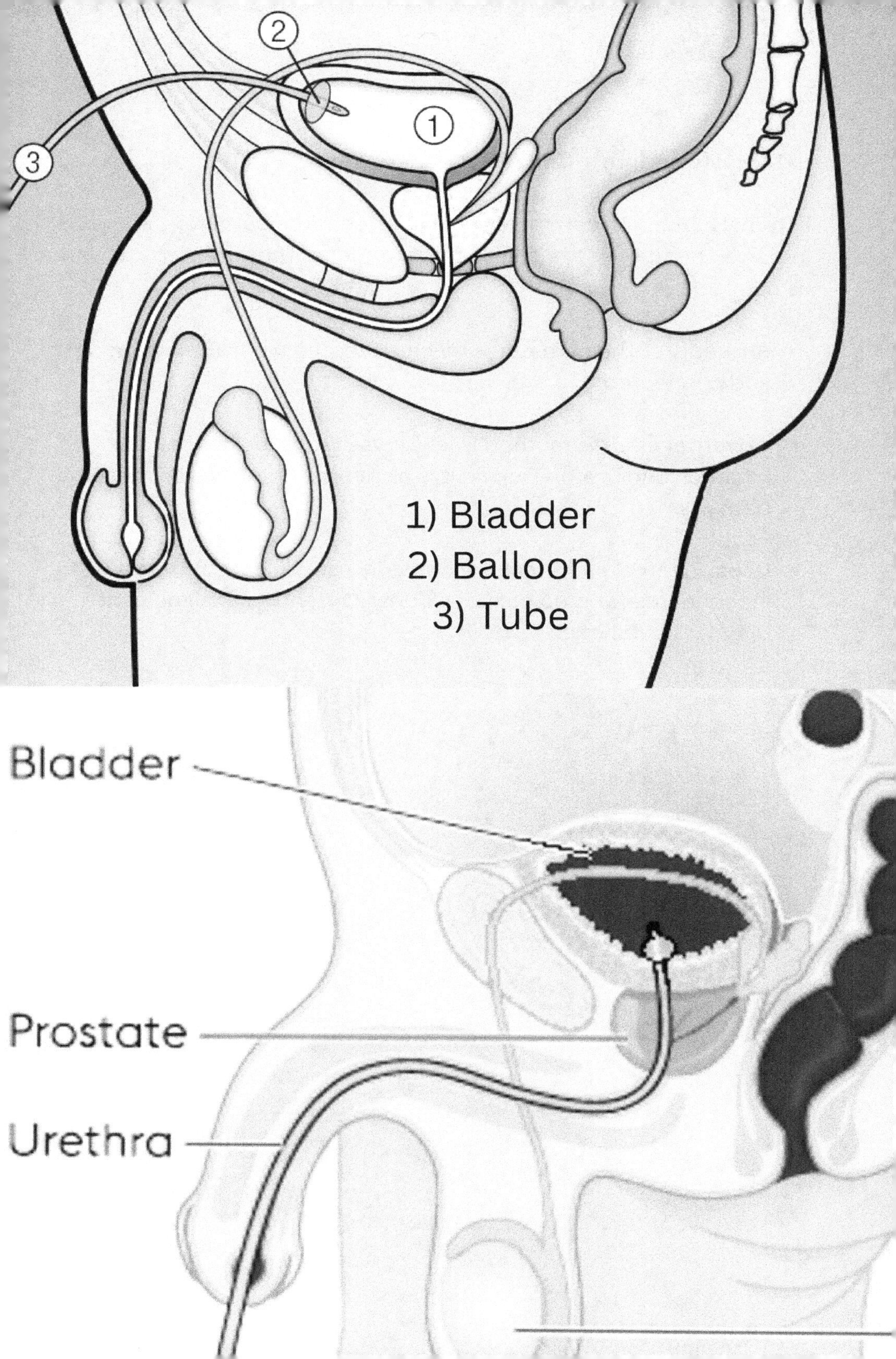
1) Bladder
2) Balloon
3) Tube
Bladder
Prostate
Urethra

External (Condom)– Conveen Catherisation

External catheters, commonly known as condom catheters, are non-invasive and fit over the penis to collect urine. They are also known as conveens.

- **Procedure:** The catheter is placed over the penis like a condom and connected to a drainage bag.

- **Advantages**: This method is less invasive, reducing the risk of infection and urethral injury. It is also more comfortable for some patients.

- **Uses:** External catheters are primarily used in male patients with incontinence who do not have urinary retention or significant bladder dysfunction.

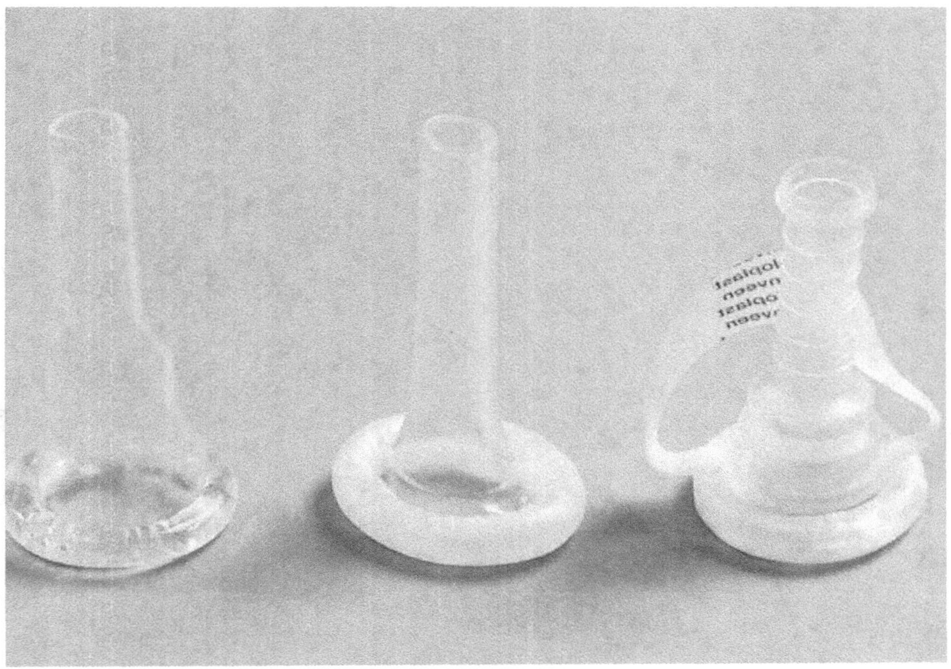

Proper Catheter Maintenance

Proper techniques for catheter maintenance are crucial to prevent complications and ensure the comfort of the care recipient.

Maintenance:

Hygiene: Regularly clean the catheter insertion site with mild soap and water. For indwelling catheters, empty the drainage bag before it becomes full and keep the bag below bladder level to prevent backflow.

Hydration: Encourage adequate fluid intake to keep urine flowing and reduce the risk of blockages.

Monitoring: Check for signs of infection, such as redness, swelling, or foul-smelling urine. Report any concerns to a healthcare provider promptly.

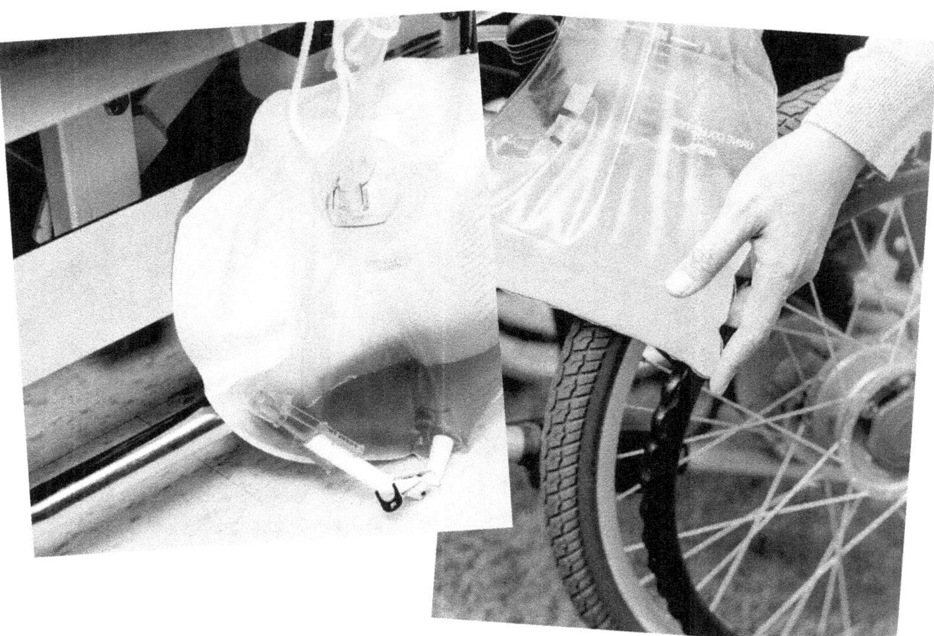

What to look for

Kinked tubing, backflow, bypassing

- Ensure that the tubing has not become kinked by pressure from patient's sitting position or clothing

- Ensure the urine collection bag is at a lower level to the patient to prevent retrograde flow

Constipation

Constipation can result in a full rectum, which can cause pressure on the drainage lumen of the catheter and stop it draining

- Ensure person maintains a good fluid intake and where appropriate offer dietary advice

- Consider use of laxatives if other measures fail

Debris and blockage

Encourage the person to maintain a good fluid intake which helps to alleviate this problem

Infection

- Check if urine is bypassing the catheter

- Check for cloudy, foul smelling urine

- Confusion or falling

- Good hygiene!

Preventing and Managing Infections and Complications

Preventing and managing infections and complications is critical for individuals using catheters. Proper hygiene and monitoring can significantly reduce these risks.

Preventing Infections:

Sterile Technique: Always use sterile techniques during catheter insertion and when handling the catheter.

Regular Cleaning: Clean the catheter and surrounding skin daily with mild soap and water.

Hydration: Encourage drinking plenty of fluids to promote regular urine flow and reduce the risk of infection. Keep a fluid chart to regularly monitor urine input and output.

Managing Complications:

Urinary Tract Infections (UTIs): Be vigilant for symptoms of UTIs, such as fever, chills, or cloudy urine. Seek medical attention promptly if these symptoms occur.

Skin Irritation: Check for signs of skin irritation or pressure sores around the catheter site. Use protective barriers and ensure the catheter is properly secured to minimize movement.

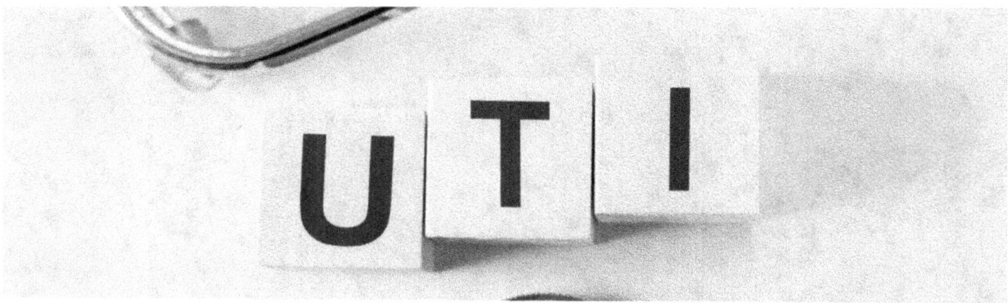

Addressing the Emotional Impact of Incontinence and Catheter Use

The emotional impact of incontinence and catheter use can be profound, affecting a man's self-esteem and mental health. Addressing these emotional aspects is as important as managing the physical care.

Empathy and Understanding: Acknowledge the embarrassment and frustration that can accompany incontinence and catheter use. Approach the subject with sensitivity and reassurance.

Open Communication: Encourage open communication about their feelings and concerns. Provide a safe space for them to express their emotions without judgment.

Maintaining Dignity: Use appropriate terminology, such as "pads" instead of "nappies" or "diapers," to maintain their dignity. Ensure privacy during all aspects of incontinence and catheter care.

Support and Encouragement: Offer emotional support and encouragement. Remind them that incontinence is a common issue and that effective management strategies are available.

Professional Support: Encourage seeking support from healthcare professionals, such as continence specialists or counsellors, who can provide additional resources and support.

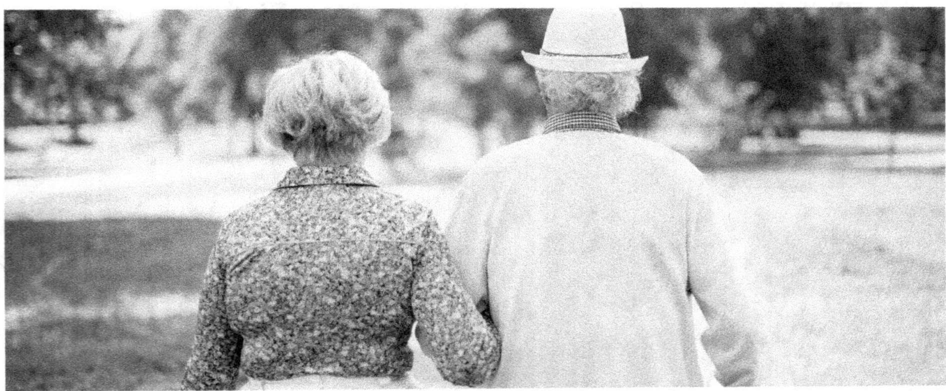

Restoring Dignity

For many patients, issues related to urinary retention or incontinence can be profoundly embarrassing and distressing. Catheterisation helps restore a sense of normalcy and dignity:

- Managing Incontinence: For patients who experience urinary incontinence, catheters offer a reliable solution that prevents the embarrassment of accidents and allows them to participate in daily activities without fear.

- Post-Surgical Recovery: After surgery, patients are often vulnerable and in discomfort. Catheterisation ensures that urinary needs are met discreetly, allowing patients to focus on recovery without additional stress.

Improving Comfort

Comfort is a critical aspect of patient care, and catheterisation can play a significant role in enhancing it:

- Relieving Discomfort: Urinary retention can cause significant pain and discomfort. By providing immediate relief, catheters improve the patient's overall sense of well-being.

- Minimizing Infections: Modern catheter designs and techniques emphasize infection prevention. Antimicrobial coatings, sterile insertion procedures, and closed drainage systems reduce the risk of catheter-associated urinary tract infections (CAUTIs), contributing to patient comfort and safety.

- Customized Care: Advances in catheter technology mean that patients can receive catheters tailored to their specific needs. From different sizes and materials to options like intermittent or indwelling catheters, customization ensures maximum comfort and effectiveness.

Conclusion

In conclusion, managing incontinence and catheter care involves understanding the types and causes of urinary incontinence, using appropriate catheters, following proper insertion and maintenance techniques, preventing infections, and addressing the emotional impact on male care recipients. By approaching these aspects with sensitivity and care, caregivers can help maintain the dignity, comfort, and overall well-being of the individuals they support.

This knowledge will further equip you to provide compassionate and competent care, ensuring that patients can go with dignity and comfort.

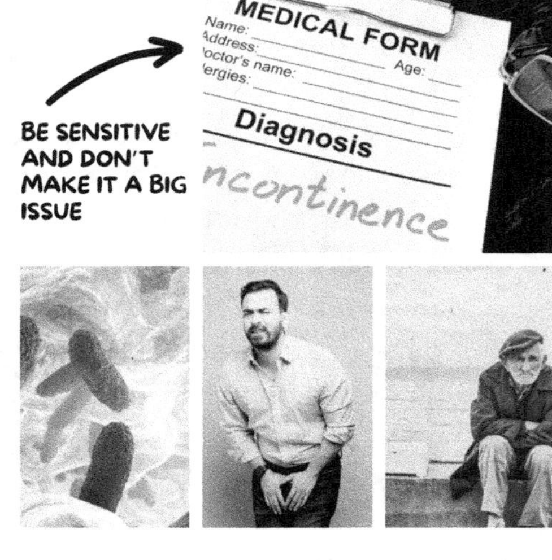

SHOW YOU CARE

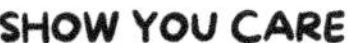

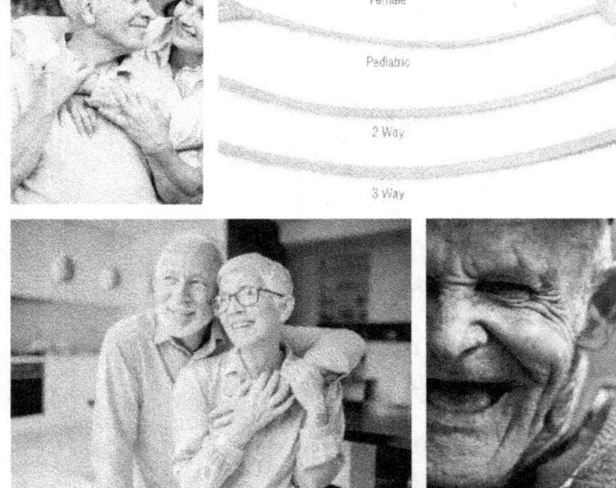

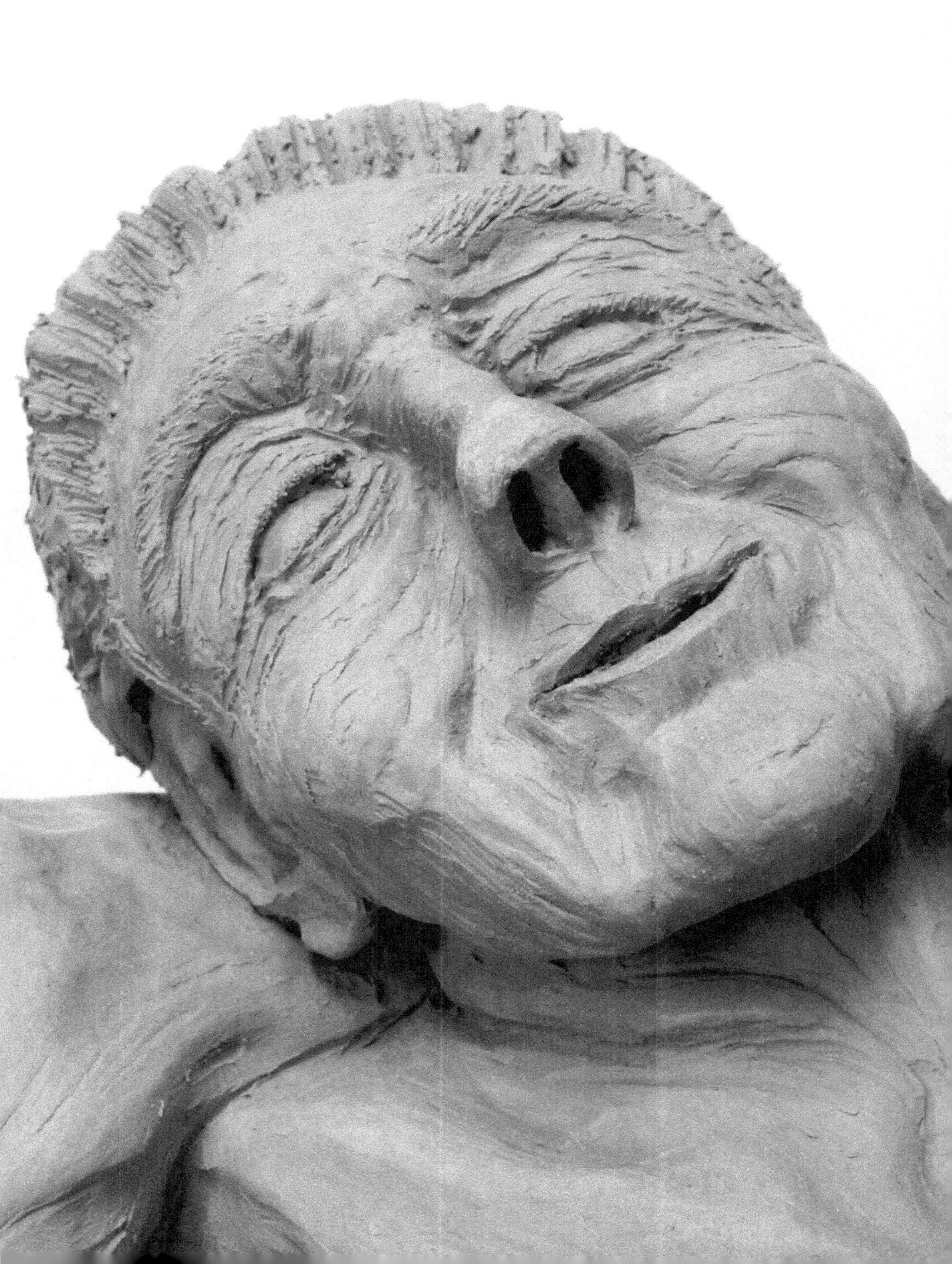

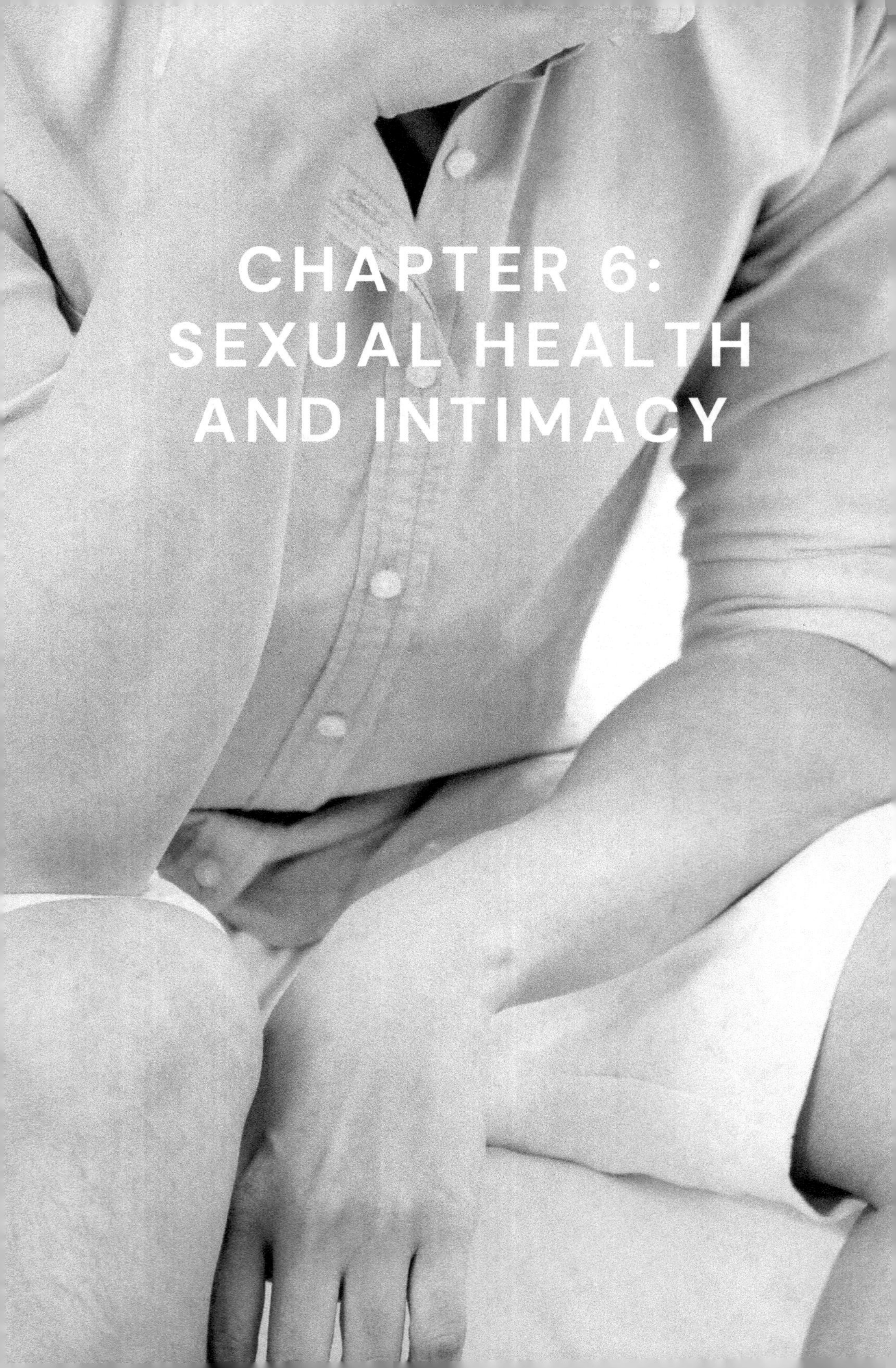

CHAPTER 6:
SEXUAL HEALTH
AND INTIMACY

Addressing Sexual Health Concerns

Sexual health and intimacy are integral aspects of overall well-being, but they can be particularly challenging topics for men receiving care. These issues can be a source of frustration and feelings of loss, as many men place a high value on their sexual health and intimate relationships. This chapter aims to address these concerns with sensitivity and professionalism.

Men may experience a range of sexual health concerns, especially as they age or face health issues. These can include erectile dysfunction (ED), reduced libido, difficulties with ejaculation, and involuntary erections.

Understanding these concerns and their underlying causes is the first step in providing effective support.

Without this understanding, this can lead to deprerssion, feelings of helplessness, embaressment and sadness.

Older generations always find this a difficult subject to talk about as their parents found it a taboo subject. It is only really in recent times that people have begun to talk about this.

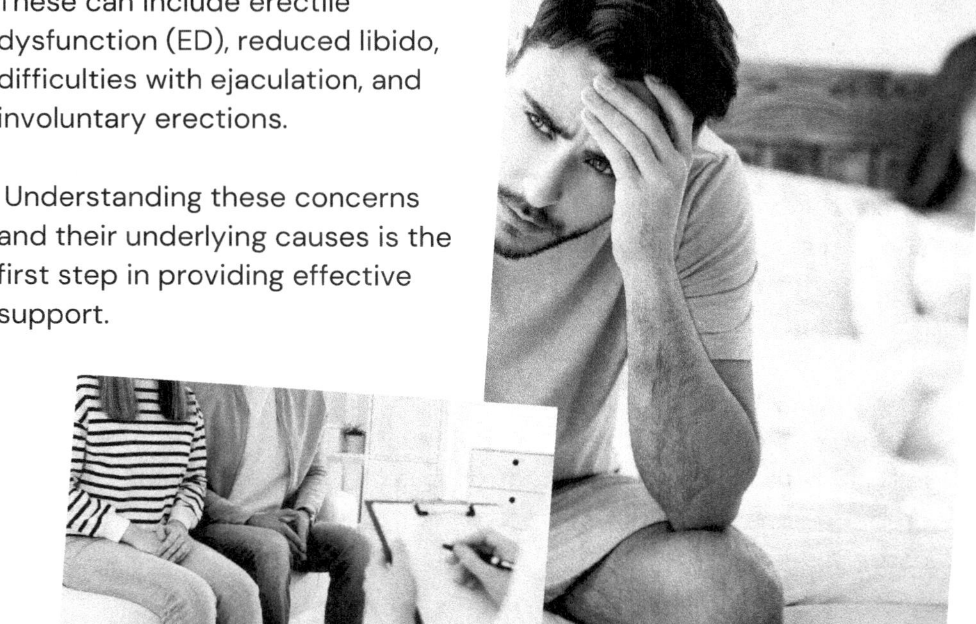

Erectile Dysfunction (ED): ED is the inability to achieve or maintain an erection sufficient for sexual activity. It can be caused by physical factors (e.g., cardiovascular disease, diabetes, obesity), psychological factors (e.g., stress, anxiety, depression), or a combination of both.

Reduced Libido: A decrease in sexual desire can result from hormonal changes, medications, chronic illnesses, or psychological issues. It's important to consider these factors when addressing concerns about libido.

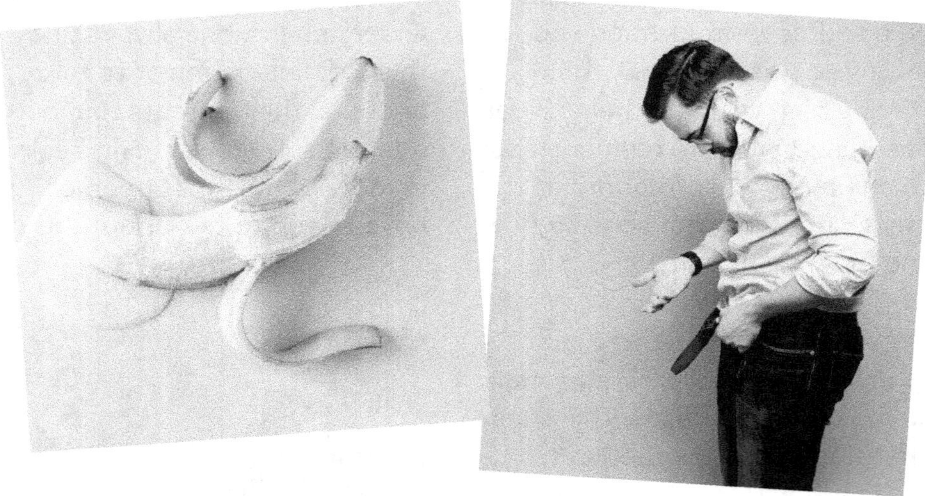

Ejaculatory Issues: These can include premature ejaculation, delayed ejaculation, or an inability to ejaculate. Some men with enlarged prostates may experience a different kind of ejaculation, where the semen struggles to get past the prostate and sometimes ends up ejaculating into the bladder, causing a strange sensation. Such issues can stem from psychological stress, medical conditions, or medications.

Involuntary Erections: Men may experience involuntary erections during personal care. These can be caused by physical stimulation and are often beyond their control. This can be a source of embarrassment and discomfort for both the care recipient and the caregiver.

Providing Support for Sexual Health Issues and ED

Providing support for sexual health issues requires a compassionate and non-judgmental approach. It's important to create an environment where men feel comfortable discussing their concerns.

Open Communication: Encourage open and honest conversations about sexual health. Assure the individual that their concerns are common and that help is available.

Medical Consultation: Recommend consulting a healthcare provider who can offer medical interventions such as medications for ED, hormone therapy, or other treatments tailored to their specific needs.

Lifestyle Changes: Advise on lifestyle changes that can improve sexual health, such as regular exercise, a balanced diet, quitting smoking, reducing alcohol intake, and managing stress.

Psychological Support: Consider referring to a therapist or counselor who specializes in sexual health to address psychological factors contributing to sexual health issues.

Navigating Conversations About Intimacy and Relationships

Conversations about intimacy and relationships can be sensitive, particularly for men who may feel uncomfortable discussing these topics.

Approach with Sensitivity: Initiate conversations in a respectful and private setting. Use open-ended questions to allow the individual to express their concerns and feelings.

Acknowledge Feelings: Validate their feelings of frustration or loss. Acknowledge that changes in sexual health and intimacy can be difficult to cope with and that these feelings are normal.

Provide Resources: Offer information and resources on maintaining intimacy and emotional connection in relationships. This can include strategies for enhancing non-sexual intimacy and communication with partners.

Encourage Partner Involvement: If appropriate, involve the partner in discussions about sexual health and intimacy. This can help in understanding and addressing concerns together, fostering a supportive environment.

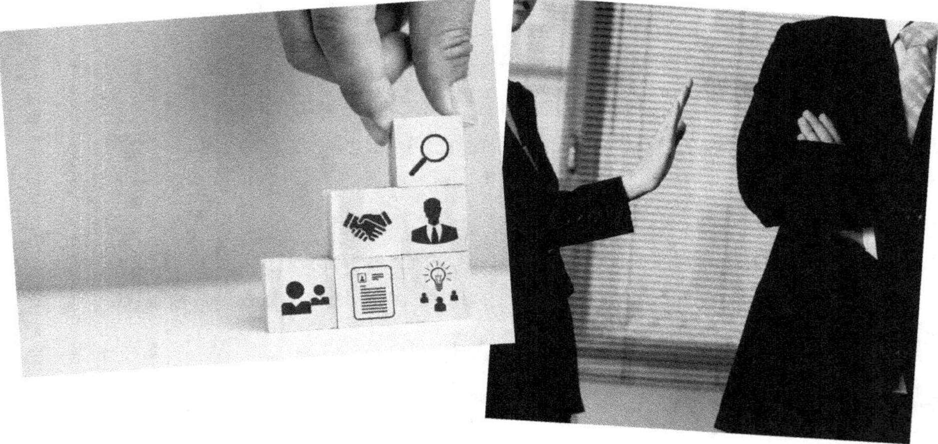

Respecting Boundaries and Maintaining Professionalism

Maintaining professionalism and respecting boundaries are crucial when addressing sexual health and intimacy.

Professional Boundaries: Clearly define and maintain professional boundaries. Avoid sharing personal opinions or experiences that may blur the caregiver-recipient relationship.

Cultural Sensitivity: Be aware of cultural and personal values related to sexual health and intimacy. Respect these values and adapt your approach accordingly.

Empathy and Respect: Always approach discussions with empathy and respect. Recognize the sensitivity of the topic and strive to create a supportive and understanding atmosphere.

Conclusion

In conclusion, addressing sexual health and intimacy in male care recipients involves understanding common concerns, providing appropriate support, navigating sensitive conversations, and maintaining professionalism.

Ensure confidentiality when discussing sexual health issues. Respect the individual's privacy and handle their information with discretion. There is nothing worst when someone thinks that you have shared personal information about them especially when it is about a mans sexual health.

By approaching these topics with sensitivity and empathy, caregivers can help men cope with their sexual health issues and maintain their dignity and quality of life.

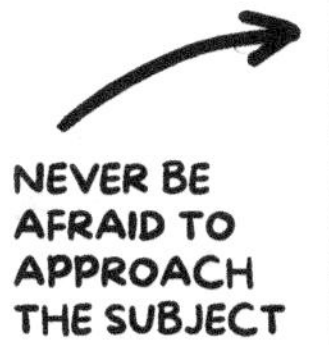

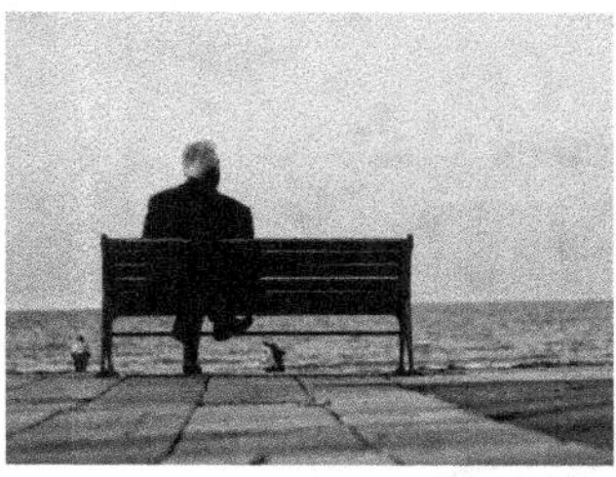

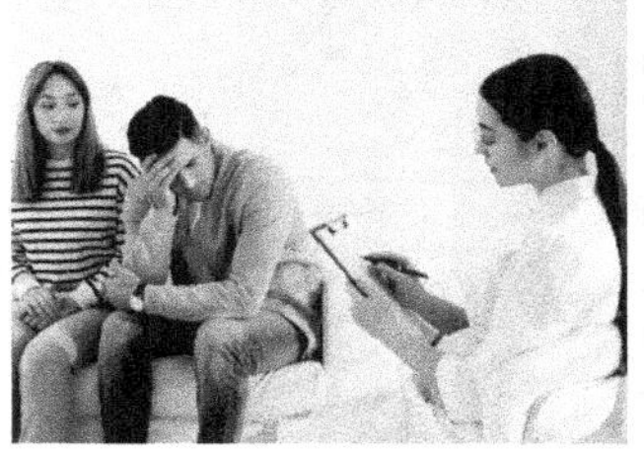

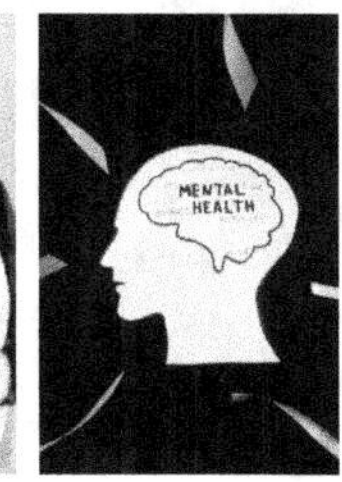

IT IS IMPORANT TO MOST MEN

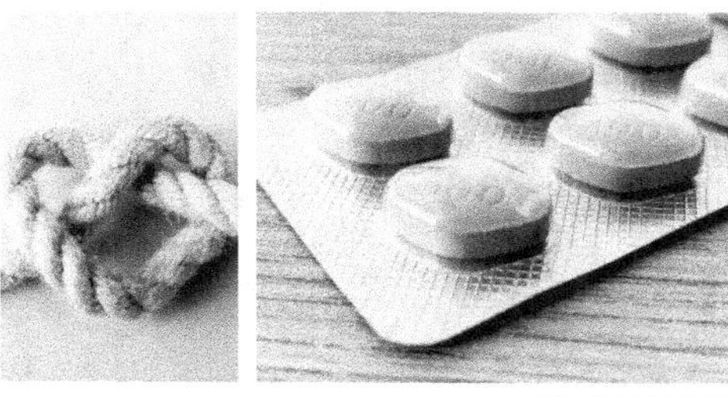

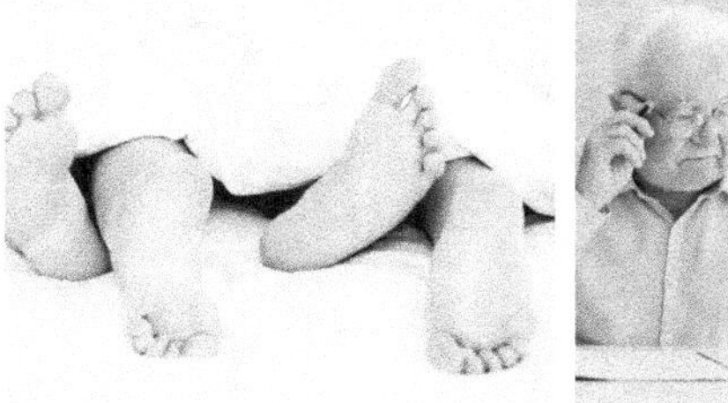

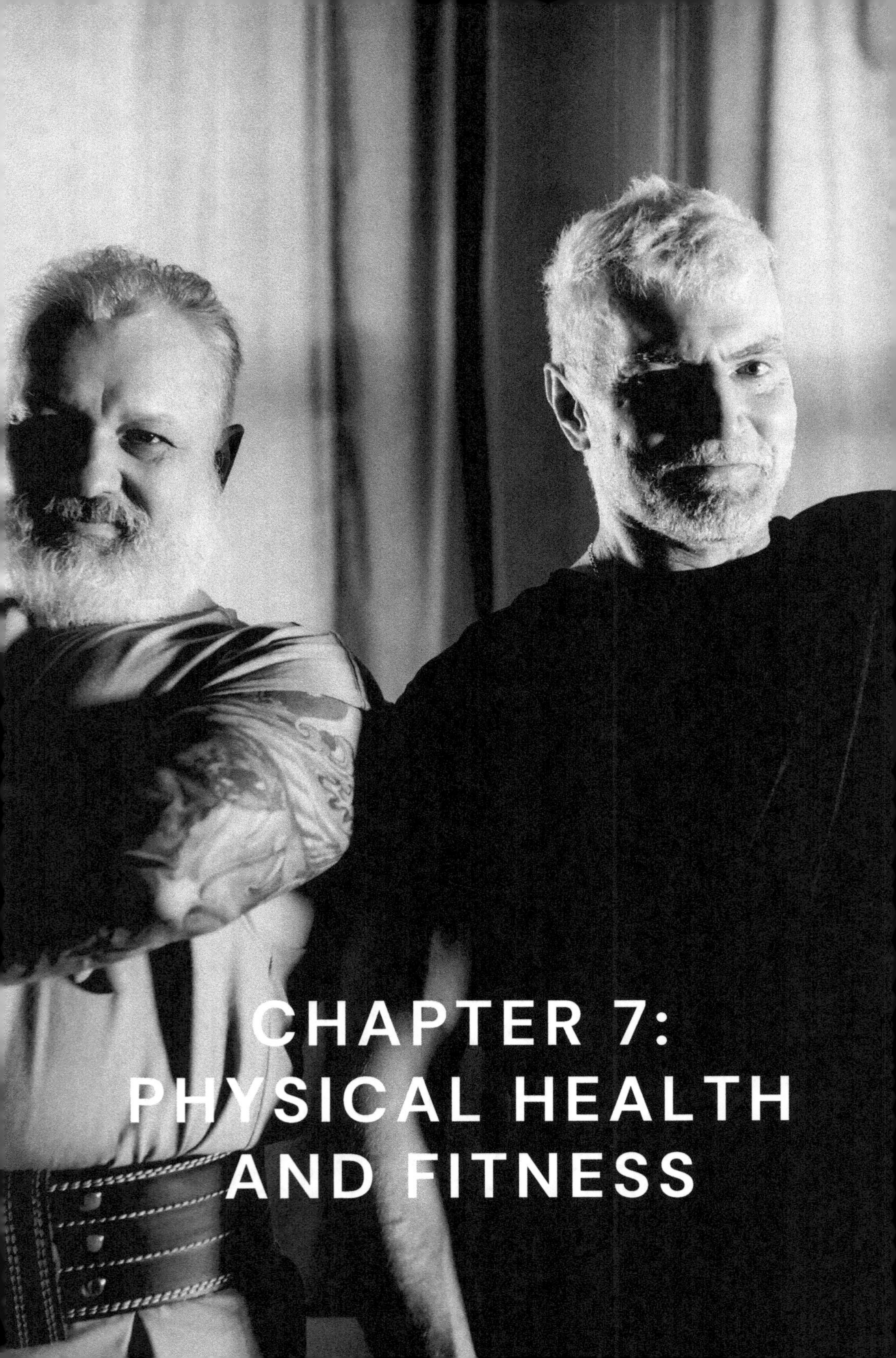
CHAPTER 7:
PHYSICAL HEALTH
AND FITNESS

Encouraging Tailored Physical Activity

Maintaining physical health and fitness is essential for overall well-being, especially for men who may face unique health challenges. Encouraging physical activity, providing safe exercise routines, monitoring chronic conditions, and offering nutritional guidance can significantly improve their quality of life. This chapter will explore these topics and emphasize the importance of involving men in their own care, including food preparation and cooking, to promote healthy eating habits.

Physical activity is crucial for maintaining strength, flexibility, and overall health. However, it's important to tailor activities to the individual's abilities and limitations to ensure safety and effectiveness.

Assessment of Abilities

Begin by assessing the individual's physical capabilities and limitations. Consider factors such as age, mobility, strength, and any existing medical conditions.

Encouragement and Motivation

Encourage the individual to stay active by highlighting the benefits of physical activity, such as improved mood, better sleep, increased energy, and enhanced mobility. Set achievable goals and celebrate progress to maintain motivation.

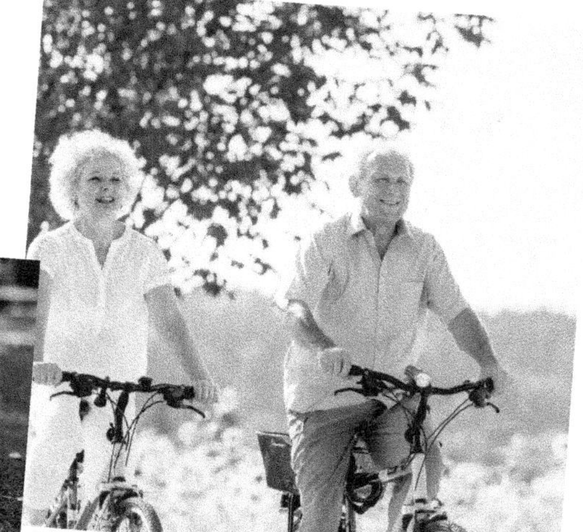

Personalized Exercise Plans.

Develop a personalized exercise plan that takes into account the individual's preferences and goals. Activities can include walking, swimming, light aerobics, or yoga, depending on what is suitable and enjoyable for them.

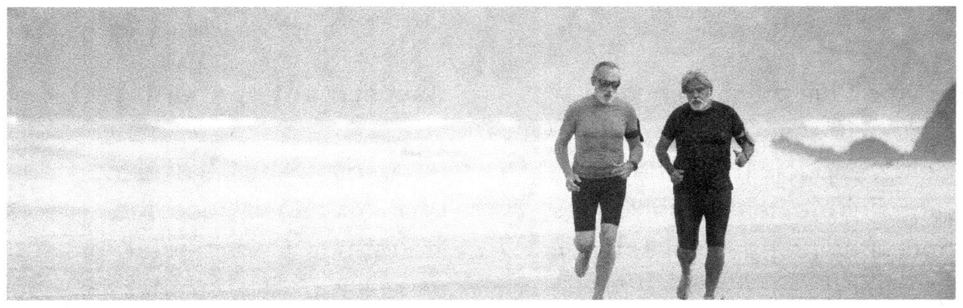

Safe Exercise Routines for Strength and Flexibility

Incorporating safe exercise routines into daily life can help maintain and improve physical health. Focus on exercises that enhance strength, flexibility, and overall fitness without causing injury.

Strength Training: Include exercises that build muscle strength, such as light weightlifting, resistance band exercises, or body-weight exercises like squats and push-ups. Ensure that exercises are performed with proper form to prevent injury.

Flexibility Exercises: Promote flexibility through stretching routines, yoga, or tai chi. These activities can help maintain range of motion, reduce stiffness, and prevent injuries.

Balance and Coordination: Incorporate exercises that improve balance and coordination, such as standing on one foot, heel-to-toe walking, or balance board exercises. These can help reduce the risk of falls.

Safety Measures: Ensure that all exercises are performed in a safe environment. Provide guidance on proper techniques and use of equipment. Supervise activities if necessary, and be mindful of any signs of overexertion or discomfort.

Monitoring and Managing Chronic Conditions

Many men may have chronic conditions such as diabetes or heart disease that require careful monitoring and management. Physical activity and proper healthcare can help control these conditions and improve overall health.

Regular Monitoring: Keep track of key health indicators, such as blood sugar levels for diabetes or blood pressure for heart disease. Regular monitoring helps in identifying any issues early and adjusting care plans accordingly.

Medication Management: Ensure that the individual takes prescribed medications as directed. Monitor for any side effects and communicate with healthcare providers to manage any concerns.

Lifestyle Modifications: Encourage lifestyle changes that can help manage chronic conditions, such as quitting smoking, reducing alcohol intake, managing stress, and maintaining a healthy weight.

Professional Support: Work with healthcare professionals to develop and follow a comprehensive care plan. Regular check-ups with doctors, dietitians, and other specialists can provide valuable support and guidance.

Nutritional Guidance for a Balanced Diet

A balanced diet is fundamental to maintaining health and managing chronic conditions. Providing nutritional guidance and involving men in food preparation can promote healthier eating habits.Educate the individual on the basics of a balanced diet, including the importance of fruits, vegetables, whole grains, lean proteins, and healthy fats. Encourage moderation in salt, sugar, and saturated fats.

Meal Planning: Assist with meal planning to ensure a variety of nutritious foods. Create meal plans that are easy to prepare and suit the individual's taste preferences and dietary needs.
Involvement in Cooking: Involve the individual in food preparation and cooking. This can foster a sense of independence and encourage them to take an active role in their health. Simple tasks like chopping vegetables, stirring ingredients, or following a recipe can be enjoyable and rewarding.

Conclusion

In conclusion, maintaining physical health and fitness through tailored physical activity, safe exercise routines, chronic condition management, and balanced nutrition is vital for men's overall well-being.

By involving men in their own care, especially in food preparation and cooking, caregivers can promote healthier lifestyles and improve the quality of life for the individuals they support.

Emphasize the importance of staying hydrated. Encourage drinking water regularly and reducing the intake of sugary drinks and excessive caffeine.

Be mindful of any special dietary needs or restrictions due to medical conditions. Consult with a dietitian for personalized advice and meal planning.

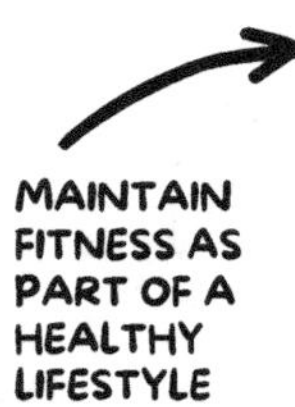

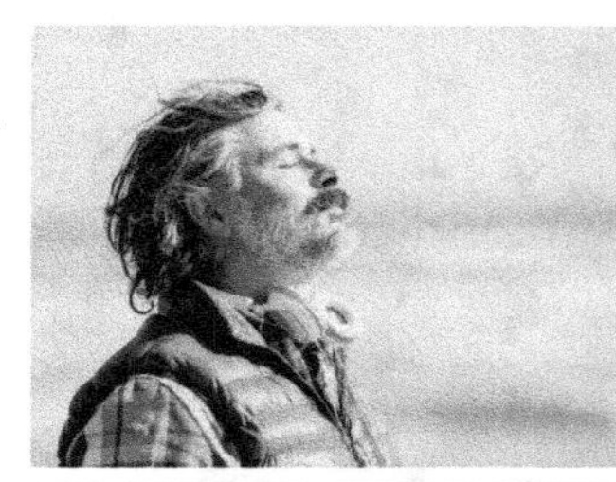

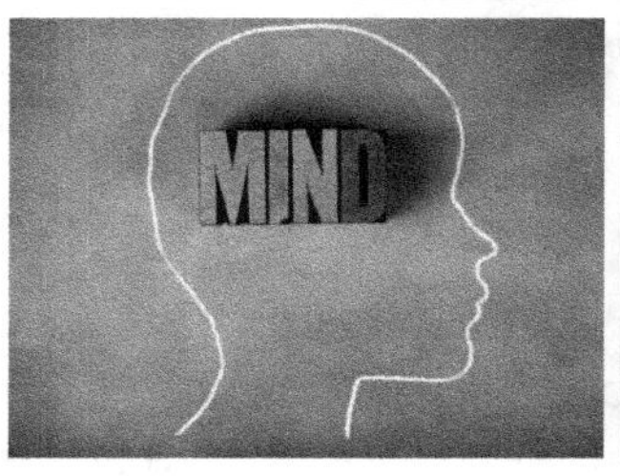

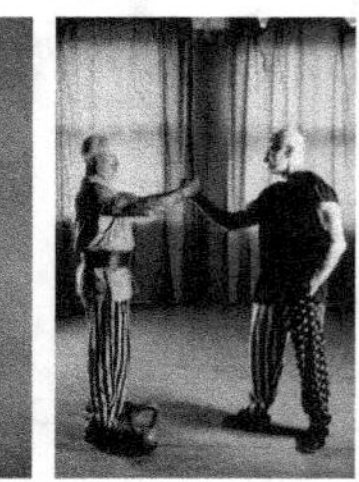

FIT BODY- FIT MIND

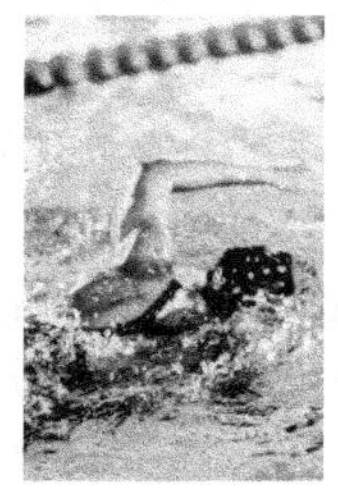

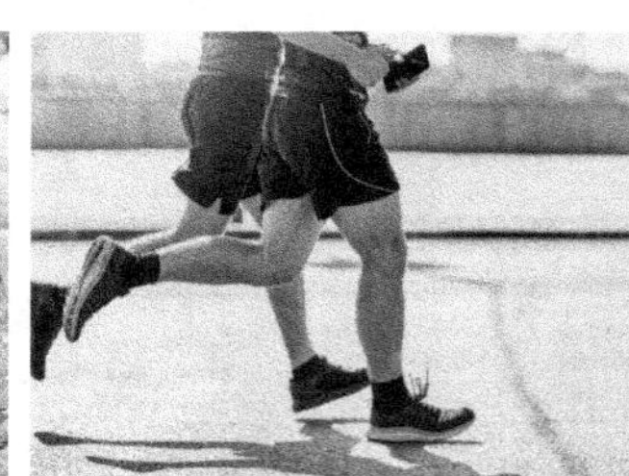

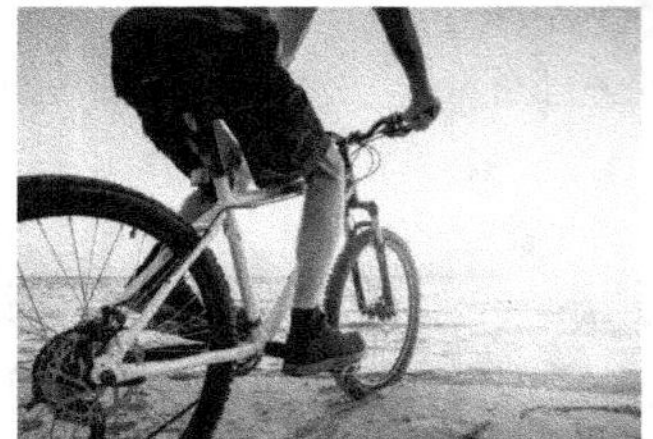

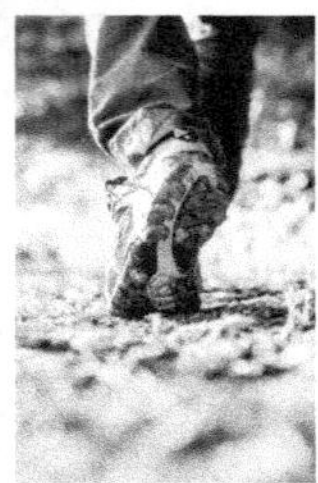

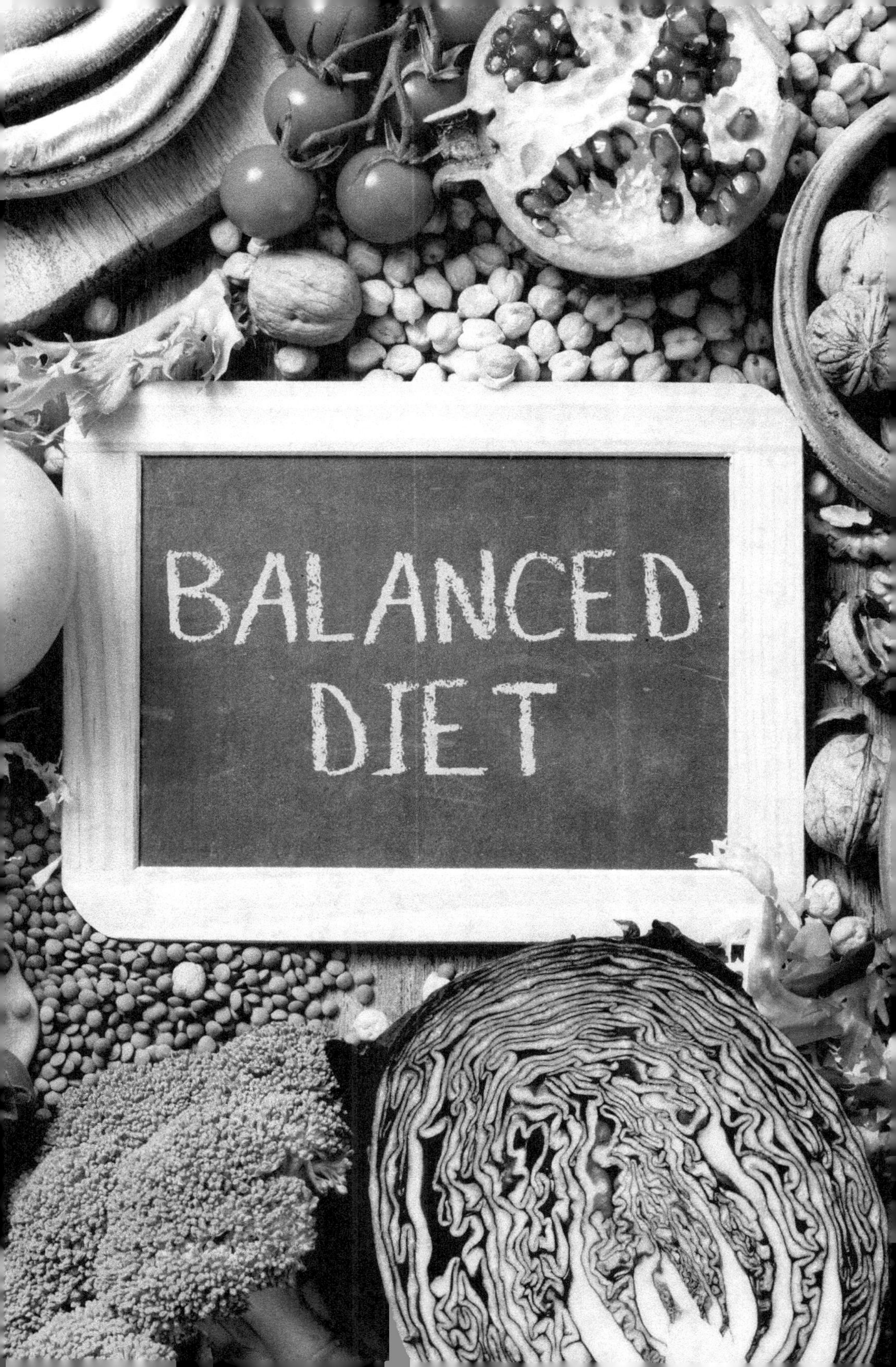

BALANCED
DIET

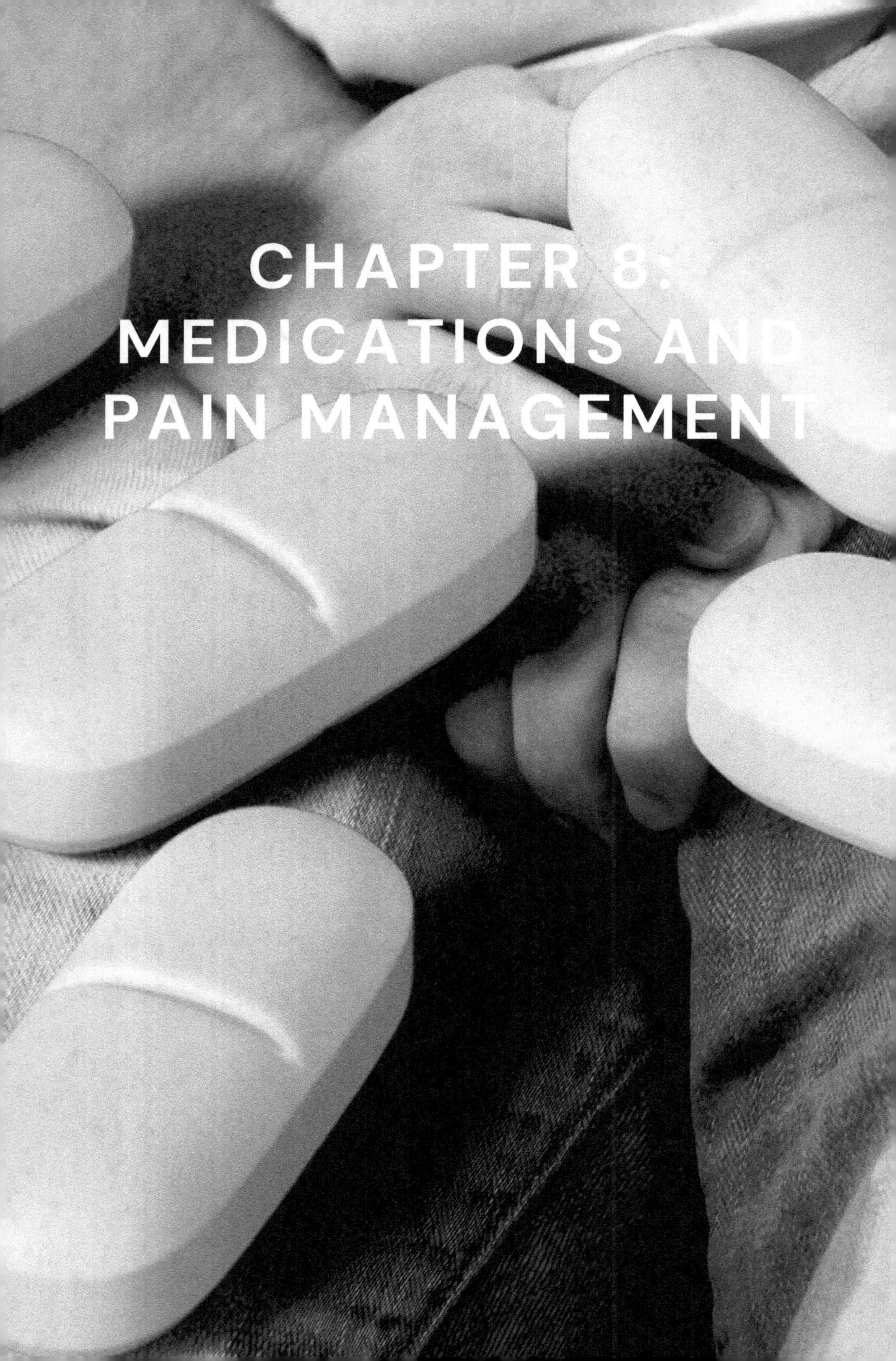
CHAPTER 8:
MEDICATIONS AND
PAIN MANAGEMENT

Understanding Common Medications for Male Health Issues

Medications and pain management are critical components of male health care. Understanding common medications, ensuring adherence, managing side effects, employing effective pain management techniques, and recognizing signs of medication misuse or abuse are essential skills for caregivers. Additionally, exploring natural remedies can offer complementary options for managing health issues.

Men often require medications to manage a variety of health conditions, from chronic diseases to acute issues. Understanding these medications helps caregivers provide better support.

Medications for Chronic Conditions: Common medications include antihypertensives for high blood pressure, statins for high cholesterol, and metformin for diabetes. These medications require regular monitoring and adherence to ensure effectiveness.

Medications for Male-Specific Issues: These include medications for prostate health, such as alpha-blockers and 5-alpha-reductase inhibitors, and treatments for erectile dysfunction (ED), such as sildenafil (Viagra) and tadalafil (Cialis).

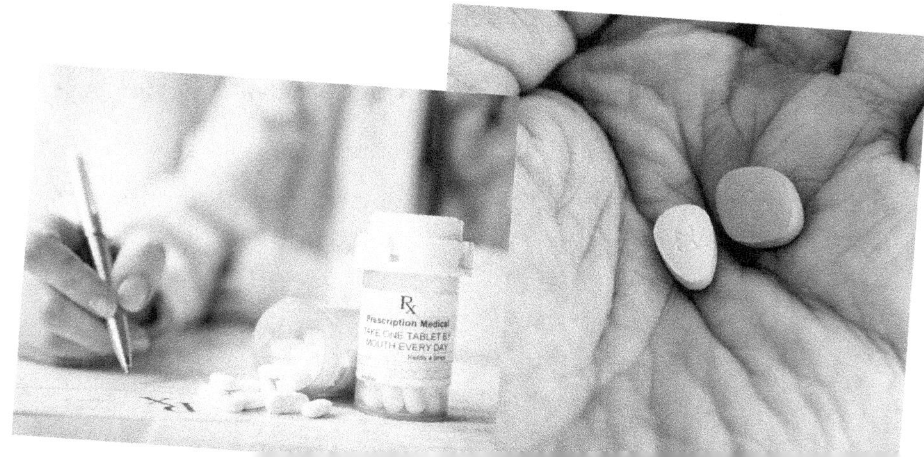

Pain Medications: Pain management may involve over-the-counter options like acetaminophen or ibuprofen, as well as prescription opioids for more severe pain. Nonsteroidal anti-inflammatory drugs (NSAIDs) are commonly used for conditions like arthritis.

Mental Health Medications: Antidepressants and anxiolytics may be prescribed for mental health conditions. Understanding their effects and side effects is crucial for providing comprehensive care.

Ensuring Medication Adherence and Managing Side Effects

Ensuring that medications are taken correctly and managing any side effects are vital for effective treatment.

Medication Adherence: Create a schedule and use pill organizers to help with adherence. Reminders via phone alarms or caregiver prompts can also be beneficial. Educate the individual on the importance of taking their medications as prescribed.

Managing Side Effects: Be aware of potential side effects for each medication. Common side effects include gastrointestinal issues, dizziness, and fatigue. Report any severe or unexpected reactions to a healthcare provider immediately.

Monitoring Effectiveness: Keep track of the individual's response to medications. Regularly review their symptoms and any changes in their condition with healthcare professionals.

Techniques for Effective Pain Management

Pain management is a critical aspect of caregiving, requiring a multi-faceted approach.

Medication Management: Use prescribed pain medications as directed. Be aware of the proper dosages and timings to avoid overuse and dependence.

Physical Therapies: Encourage physical therapies such as massage, physiotherapy, and gentle exercises that can help alleviate pain and improve mobility.

Cognitive Behavioural Techniques: Techniques such as mindfulness, relaxation exercises, and cognitive behavioural therapy (CBT) can be effective in managing chronic pain and reducing stress.

Natural Remedies: Consider natural remedies such as herbal supplements (e.g., turmeric for its anti-inflammatory properties), acupuncture, and essential oils. Always consult with a healthcare provider before starting any new treatment to ensure it is safe and appropriate.

Recognizing Signs of Medication Misuse or Abuse

Medication misuse or abuse can have serious consequences. It's important to recognize the signs and take appropriate action.

Identifying Misuse: Look for signs such as taking higher doses than prescribed, frequent requests for refills, or using medications for non-medical reasons (e.g., to relieve stress or improve mood).

Behavioural Changes: Notice any changes in behaviour such as increased secrecy, withdrawal from social interactions, or sudden mood swings.

Physical Symptoms: Be aware of physical signs such as drowsiness, confusion, slurred speech, or poor coordination, which may indicate misuse or overdose.

Intervention and Support: If you suspect medication misuse or abuse, discuss your concerns with a healthcare provider. They can offer guidance on the appropriate steps to take, which may include adjusting medications, providing counselling, or seeking addiction treatment.

Conclusion

In conclusion, managing medications and pain effectively requires a comprehensive understanding of common medications, ensuring adherence, managing side effects, employing various pain management techniques, and recognizing signs of misuse or abuse. Incorporating natural remedies can provide additional options for managing health issues. For instance, holistic approaches like acupuncture can alleviate chronic pain, yoga and meditation can reduce stress and improve mental health, and herbal supplements such as turmeric and ginger can offer anti-inflammatory benefits.

By adopting a holistic approach to medication and pain management, caregivers can significantly improve the well-being and quality of life of the men they support.

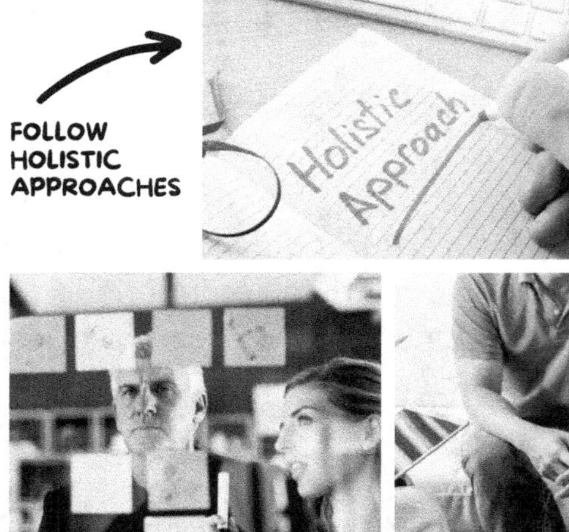

MANAGE YOUR HEALTH

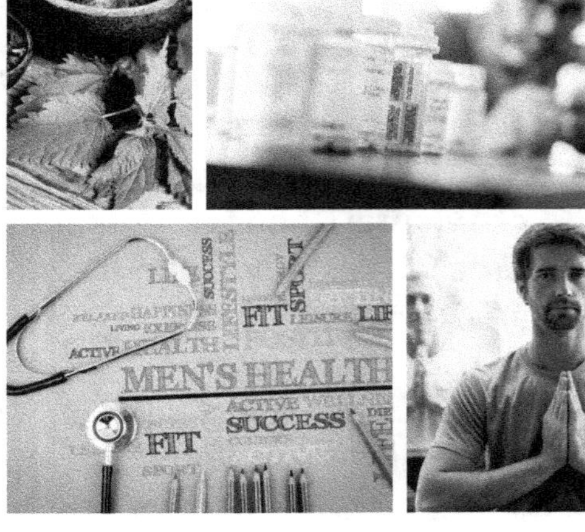

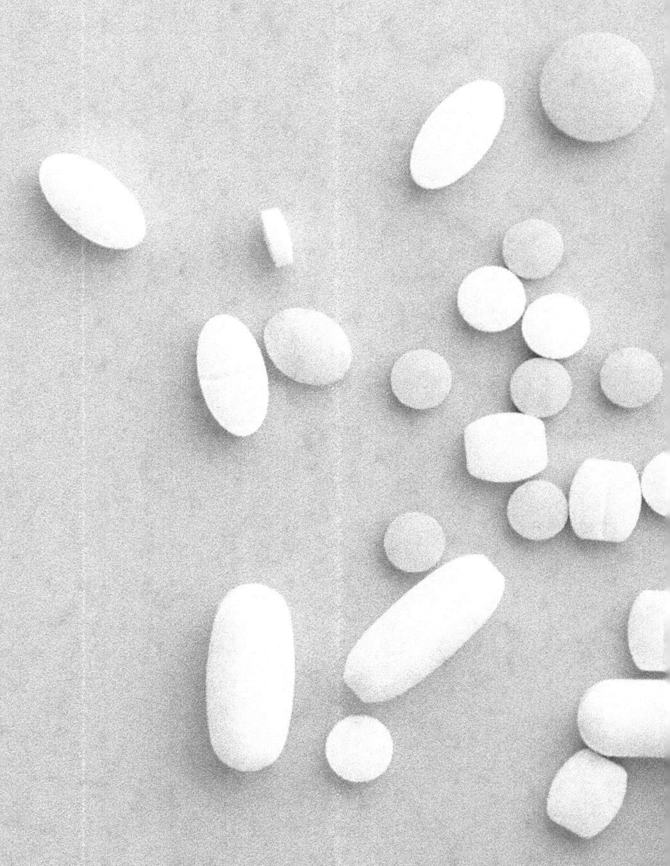

"The best form of medication is the care that you give someone and seeing them as a person"

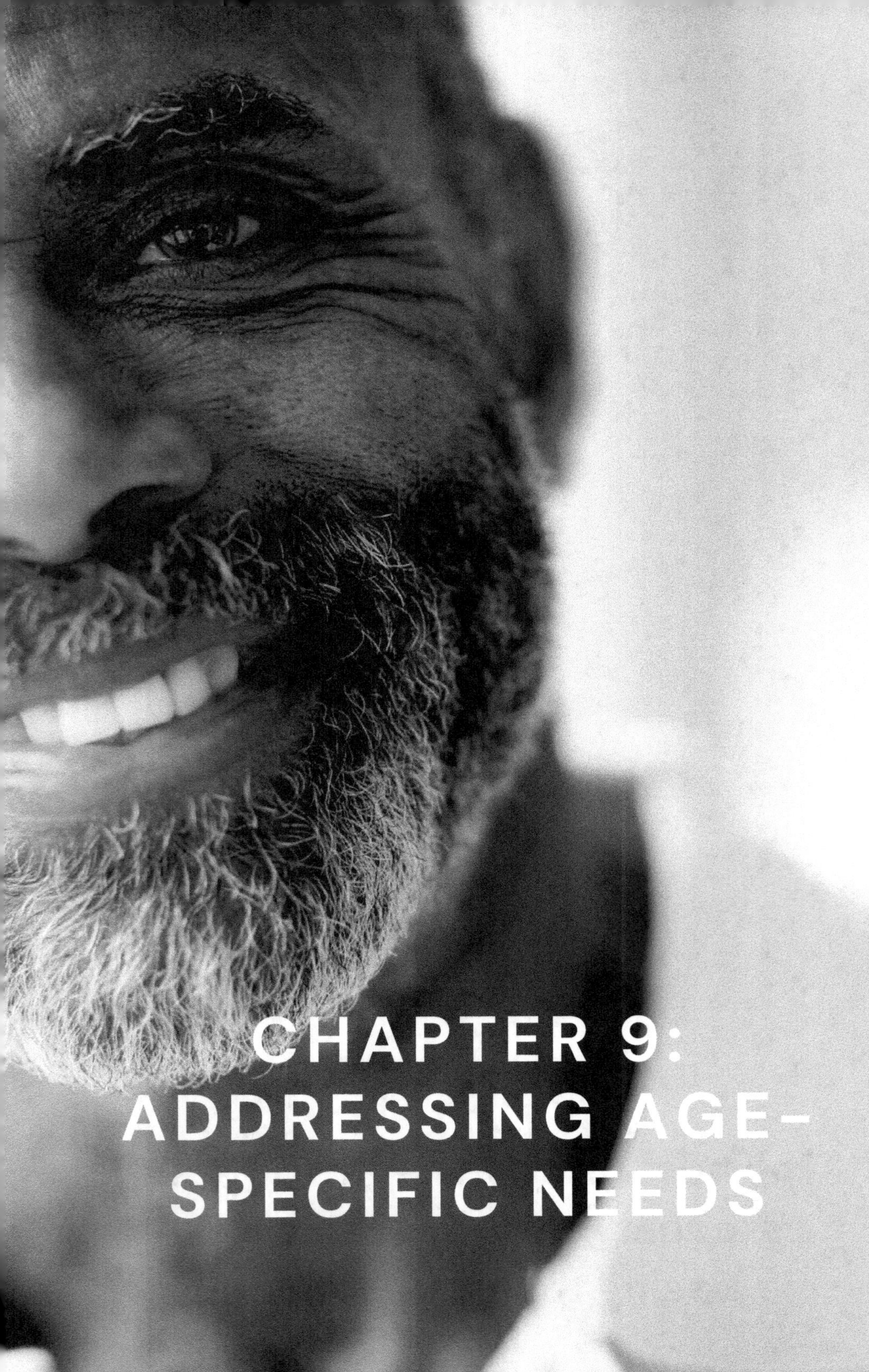

CHAPTER 9:
ADDRESSING AGE-
SPECIFIC NEEDS

Care Considerations for Elderly Male Recipients

As men age, their care needs evolve and require special attention to ensure their health, comfort, and quality of life. This chapter addresses the specific considerations for elderly male recipients, including managing age-related conditions, prostate health, supporting cognitive health, and promoting independence.

Caring for elderly men involves understanding and addressing their unique physical, emotional, and social needs.

Personalized Care Plans: Develop individualized care plans that consider the man's medical history, preferences, and daily routines. This ensures that care is tailored to his specific needs and enhances his overall well-being.

Physical Comfort: Pay attention to comfort measures, such as proper bedding, appropriate room temperature, and comfortable clothing. Regularly assess for pain and discomfort, and adjust care practices accordingly.

Emotional Support: Provide emotional support through regular communication, social interactions, and activities that the individual enjoys. Encourage participation in hobbies and interests to maintain a sense of purpose and engagement.

Social Connections: Facilitate social connections with family, friends, and community groups. Loneliness and social isolation can significantly impact mental and physical health, so maintaining these connections is crucial.

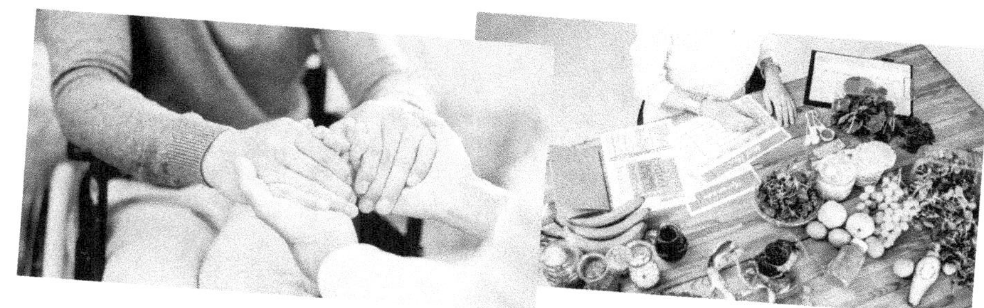

Managing Age-Related Conditions

Age-related conditions are common among elderly men and require careful management to maintain their health and quality of life.

Arthritis: Arthritis can cause pain, stiffness, and reduced mobility. Management strategies include medication, physical therapy, and exercises to improve joint function and flexibility. Heat and cold treatments can also provide relief from symptoms.

Cardiovascular Health: Monitor and manage heart health through regular check-ups, medications, and lifestyle changes such as a healthy diet and regular exercise. Encourage activities that promote cardiovascular health, such as walking and swimming.

Diabetes: For men with diabetes, careful monitoring of blood sugar levels, adherence to medication, and a balanced diet are essential. Educate about the importance of foot care and regular eye exams to prevent complications.

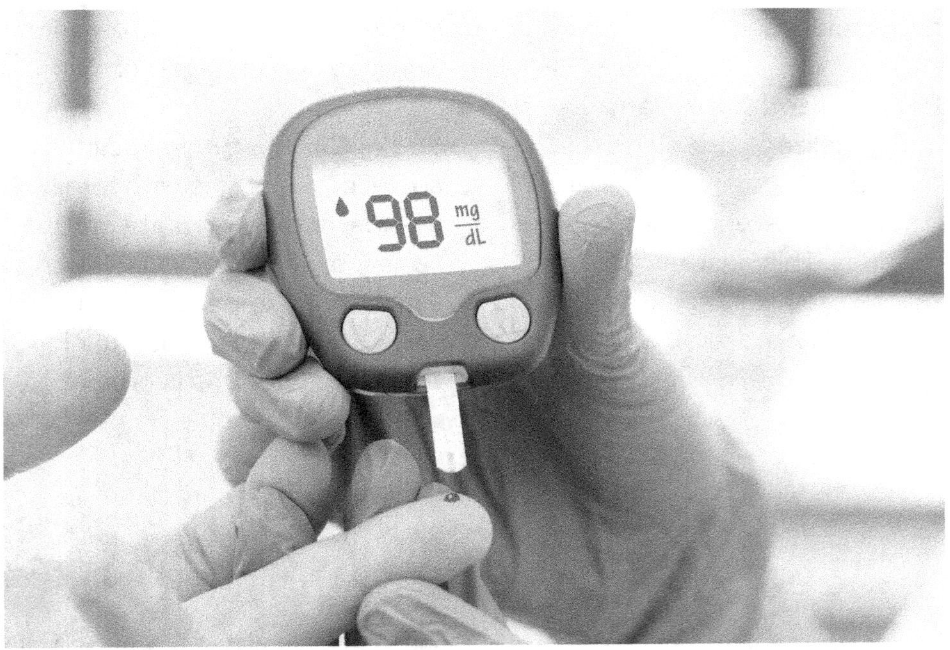

Prostate Conditions

Prostate health is a significant concern for elderly men. Understanding how to manage prostate conditions is vital for providing effective care.

Signs and Symptoms of an Enlarged Prostate: Benign Prostatic Hyperplasia (BPH) is a common condition where the prostate enlarges. Symptoms include:

- Frequent need to urinate, especially at night
- Difficulty starting urination
- Weak or interrupted urine stream
- Inability to completely empty the bladder
- Dribbling at the end of urination
- Urinary tract infections due to incomplete bladder emptying

Treatment for an Enlarged Prostate: Treatment options for BPH include:

Medications: Alpha-blockers (e.g., tamsulosin, alfuzosin) relax the muscles of the bladder neck and prostate, making it easier to urinate. 5-alpha-reductase inhibitors (e.g., finasteride, dutasteride) reduce the size of the prostate by blocking the hormone that causes prostate growth.

Minimally Invasive Procedures: Techniques such as transurethral microwave thermotherapy (TUMT) and transurethral needle ablation (TUNA) can reduce prostate tissue and improve urine flow.

Surgery: In severe cases, surgical options like transurethral resection of the prostate (TURP) or laser therapy may be necessary to remove part of the prostate.

Prostate Cancer: Regular screenings for prostate cancer are important for early detection and treatment. Educate about the symptoms, which can include difficulty urinating, blood in urine or semen, and discomfort in the pelvic area. Encourage discussions with healthcare providers regarding screening options.

Prostatitis: Prostatitis, or inflammation of the prostate, can cause pain and urinary issues. Treatment typically involves antibiotics, pain management, and sometimes physical therapy. Symptoms may include painful urination, pelvic pain, and flu-like symptoms.

Supporting Cognitive Health and Dementia Care

Cognitive health is a critical aspect of care for elderly men, particularly for those with dementia or other cognitive impairments.

Early Detection: Recognize the early signs of cognitive decline, such as memory loss, confusion, and changes in behaviour. Early detection allows for timely interventions and support.

Cognitive Stimulation: Engage in activities that stimulate the mind, such as puzzles, reading, and memory games. Social interactions and lifelong learning can also help maintain cognitive function.

Dementia Care: For those with dementia, create a safe and supportive environment. Use clear communication, establish routines, and provide reassurance to reduce anxiety and confusion. Tailor activities to the individual's abilities and interests.

Promoting Independence and Quality of Life

Maintaining independence and enhancing quality of life are central goals in caring for elderly men.

Adaptive Equipment: Utilize adaptive equipment such as grab bars, walkers, and raised toilet seats to support independence in daily activities.

Encouraging Participation: Involve the individual in decision-making and care activities as much as possible. Encourage participation in tasks they can manage, which fosters a sense of control and self-worth.

Physical Activity: Promote regular physical activity suited to their abilities. Exercise helps maintain strength, balance, and mobility, which are crucial for independence.

Nutrition and Hydration: Ensure a balanced diet and adequate hydration. Nutritional needs can change with age, so tailor the diet to meet these needs and involve the individual in meal planning and preparation.

Emotional Well-being: Address emotional well-being by providing companionship, listening to concerns, and encouraging positive activities. Support groups and counselling can also be beneficial.

Conclusion

In conclusion, addressing age-specific needs in elderly male care recipients involves understanding their unique physical and emotional challenges, managing chronic and age-related conditions, supporting cognitive health, and promoting independence and quality of life. Awareness of prostate conditions, their symptoms, and appropriate treatments is essential, as these issues can significantly affect a man's mental health and overall well-being.

By adopting a comprehensive and personalized approach, caregivers can significantly enhance the well-being and happiness of elderly men, helping them to maintain their dignity, independence, and quality of life.

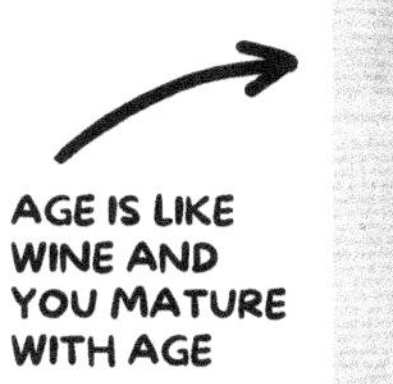

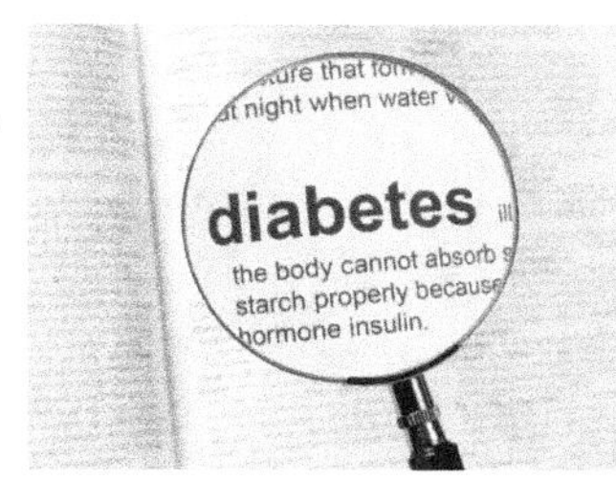

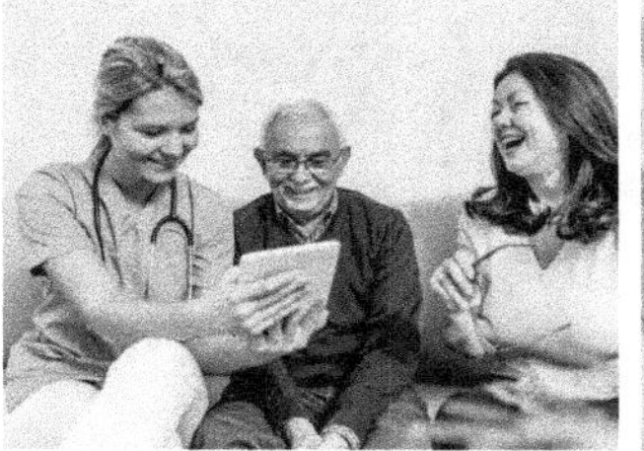
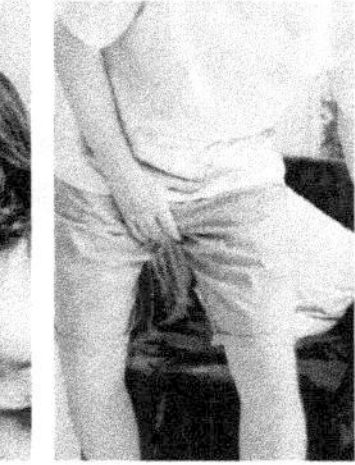

BUT AGE CAN BE SENSITIVE

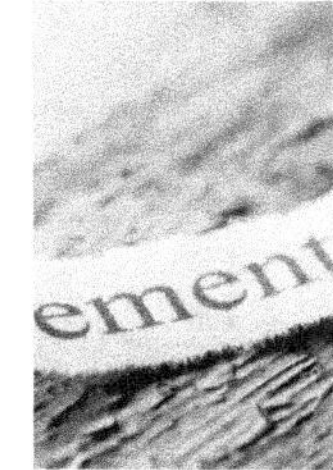

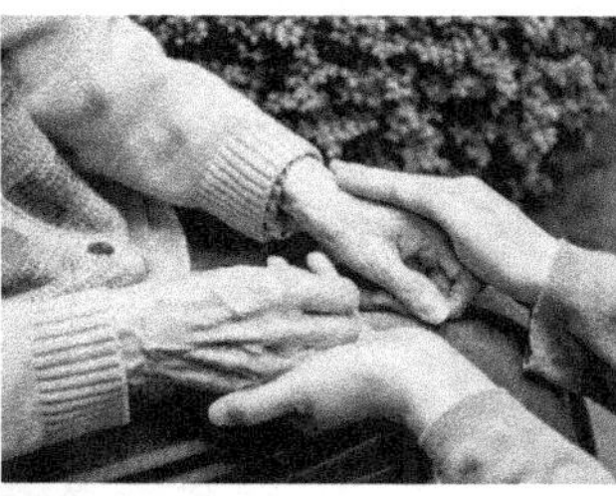

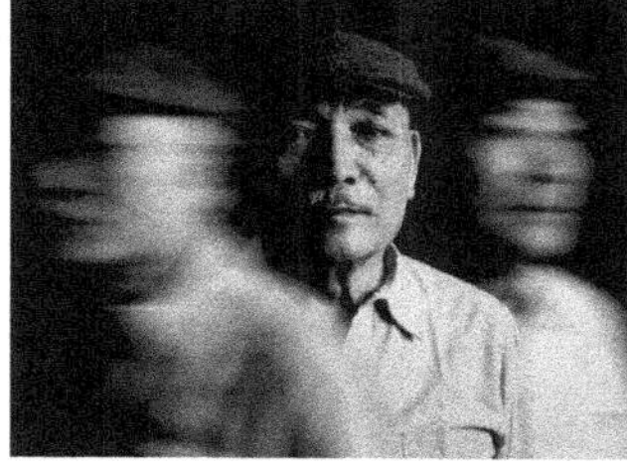
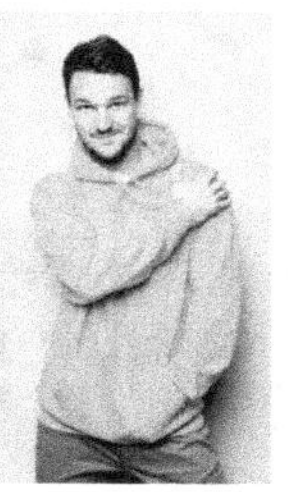

CHAPTER 10: CREATING A SAFE AND COMFORTABLE ENVIRONMENT

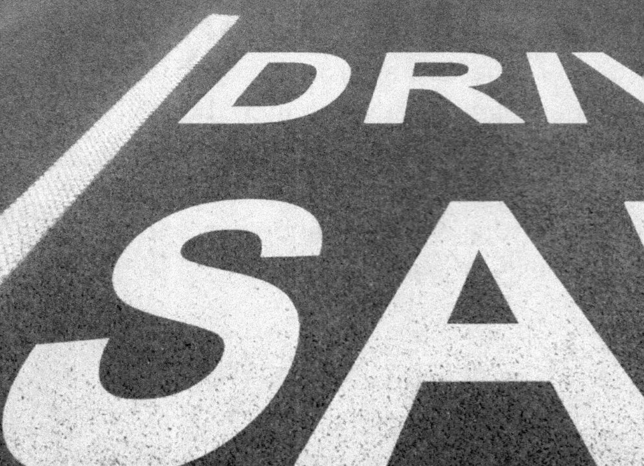

Adapting the Home to Meet the Physical Needs

Creating a safe and comfortable environment is essential for the well-being of male care recipients. This chapter focuses on adapting the home to meet physical needs, ensuring accessibility and safety, using assistive devices and technology effectively, and maintaining a clean and organized living space.

Adapting the home environment can greatly enhance the comfort and safety of male care recipients.

Mobility Aids: Install ramps or lifts to navigate stairs, and ensure doorways are wide enough for wheelchairs or walkers. Provide sturdy handrails along hallways and in frequently used areas.

Furniture Arrangement: Arrange furniture to allow for easy movement. Ensure pathways are clear and free of obstacles to prevent trips and falls.

Comfortable Seating: Provide comfortable and supportive seating options, such as recliners or chairs with armrests, to help with sitting and standing.

Lighting: Ensure adequate lighting throughout the home, including night lights in hallways and bathrooms. Use bright, non-glare lighting to reduce eye strain and improve visibility.

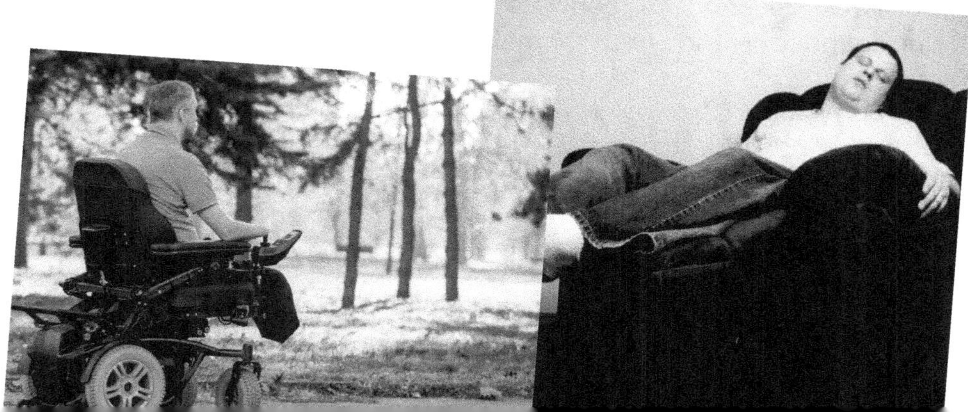

Ensuring Accessibility and Safety in the Bathroom and Living Areas

The bathroom and living areas are common places where accidents can occur. Making these areas safe and accessible is crucial.

Bathroom Safety:

Non-Slip Surfaces: Use non-slip mats in the shower and bathtub. Consider applying non-slip coatings to the bathroom floor.

Shower Chairs and Raised Toilet Seats: Provide a shower chair to allow for seated bathing. A raised toilet seat can make it easier to sit down and stand up.

Accessible Shower: Consider installing a walk-in shower with a handheld showerhead for ease of use.

Living Area Safety:

Clear Pathways: Keep pathways clear of clutter and electrical cords to prevent trips and falls.

Stable Furniture: Ensure that furniture is stable and does not tip over easily. Secure heavy items that could potentially fall.

Emergency Accessibility: Place a phone or emergency alert system within easy reach. Ensure that emergency contact information is readily available.

Using Assistive Devices and Technology Effectively

Assistive devices and technology can greatly enhance the independence and safety of male care recipients.

Mobility Aids: Use walkers, canes, or wheelchairs as needed. Ensure that the individual is trained in the proper use of these devices.

Hearing and Vision Aids: Provide hearing aids and ensure regular maintenance. Use magnifying glasses or other vision aids to assist with reading and other tasks.

Smart Home Technology: Utilize smart home devices such as voice-activated assistants to control lighting, temperature, and security systems. Automated medication dispensers can help with medication adherence.

Communication Devices: Provide easy-to-use communication devices, such as simplified phones or tablets with large buttons and screens, to stay in touch with family and caregivers.

Maintaining a Clean and Organized Living Space

A clean and organized living space contributes to a safe and comfortable environment.

Regular Cleaning: Establish a regular cleaning routine to keep the living space free of dust, dirt, and allergens. Pay special attention to high-touch areas such as doorknobs and light switches.

Decluttering: Regularly declutter to remove unnecessary items that could pose tripping hazards. Organize belongings in a way that makes them easily accessible.

Safe Storage: Store cleaning supplies, medications, and other potentially hazardous items out of reach or in locked cabinets.

Pest Control: Implement pest control measures to prevent infestations. Ensure that food is stored properly and that trash is disposed of regularly.

Air Quality: Maintain good air quality by using air purifiers and ensuring proper ventilation. Avoid using strong chemicals or fragrances that could irritate respiratory conditions.

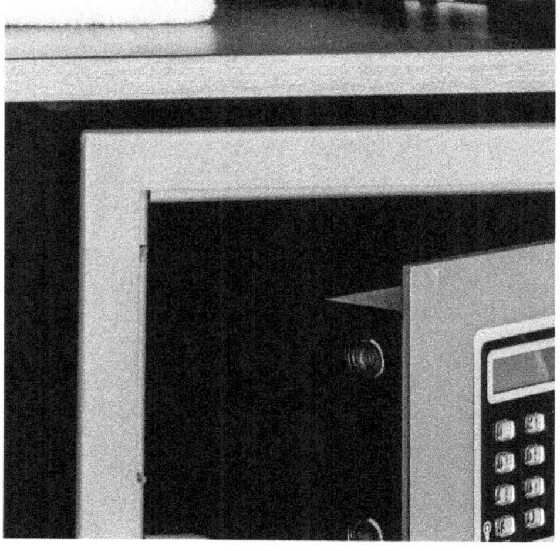

Conclusion

Creating a safe and comfortable environment for male care recipients involves adapting the home to meet their physical needs, ensuring accessibility and safety, effectively using assistive devices and technology, and maintaining a clean and organized living space. By addressing these aspects, caregivers can significantly enhance the quality of life and independence of the men they support.

A safe and comfortable environment not only prevents accidents and injuries but also promotes mental well-being and dignity, contributing to a more positive caregiving experience for both the caregiver and the care recipient.

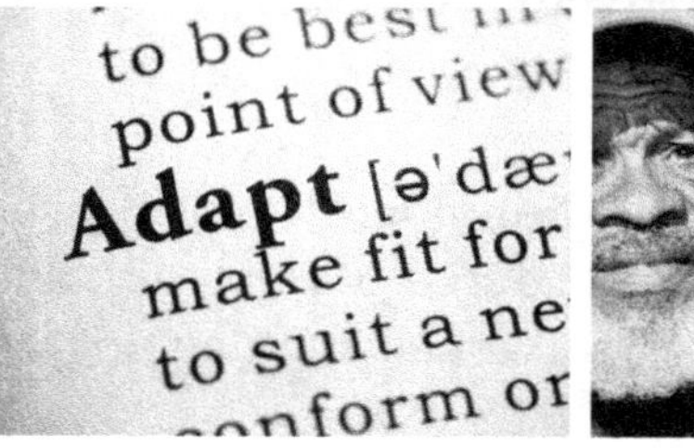

IMPROVES QULAITY OF LIFE

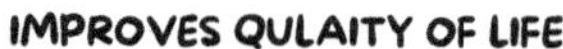

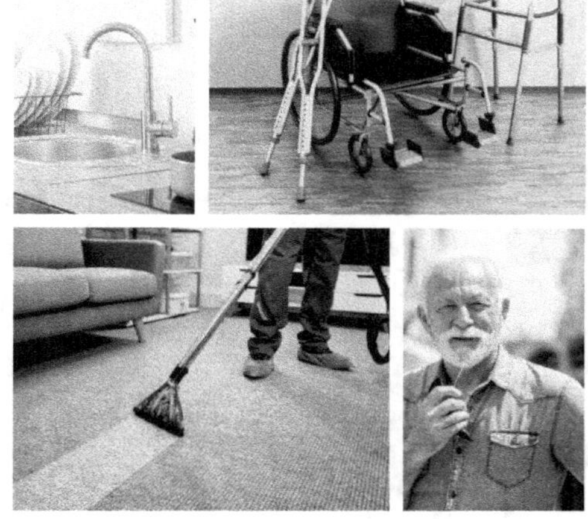

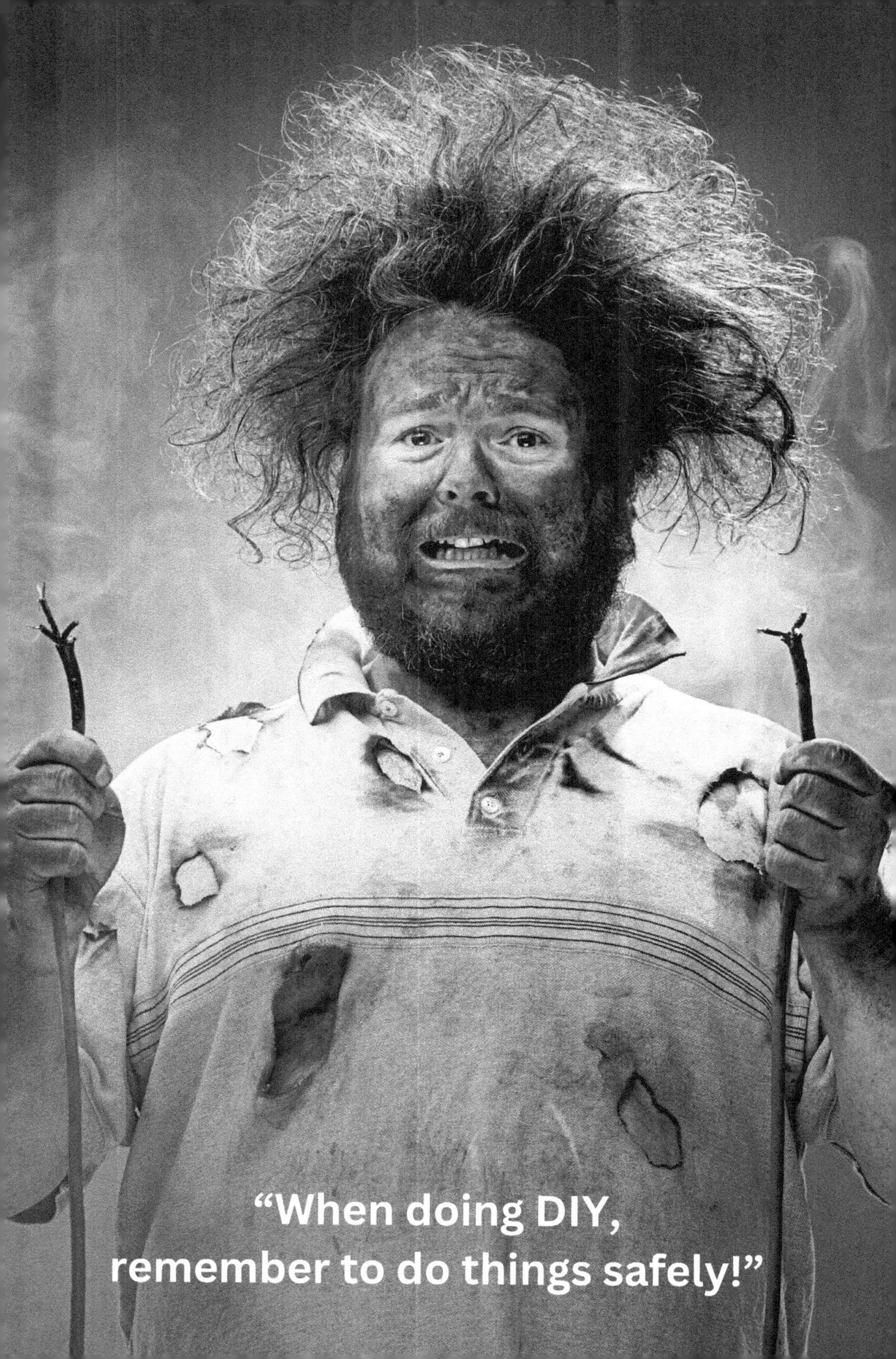
"When doing DIY,
remember to do things safely!"

CHAPTER 11: SELF-CARE FOR CARERS

Recognizing and Addressing Caregiver Burnout

Caring for others is a rewarding but demanding role that can take a toll on your physical and mental health. To provide the best care possible, it's essential to prioritize your own well-being. This chapter focuses on recognizing and addressing caregiver burnout, strategies for maintaining your health, seeking support, and balancing caregiving responsibilities with personal life.

Caregiver burnout is a state of physical, emotional, and mental exhaustion that can occur when you neglect your own needs while caring for others.

Signs of Burnout:

- Physical exhaustion and fatigue
- Emotional overwhelm or frequent irritability
- Difficulty sleeping or changes in appetite
- Loss of interest in activities you once enjoyed
- Feelings of hopelessness or depression

Addressing Burnout:

Acknowledge Your Feelings: It's important to recognize when you're feeling overwhelmed and accept that it's okay to need help.

Set Realistic Goals: Break tasks into smaller, manageable steps and set achievable goals to avoid feeling overwhelmed.

Delegate Responsibilities: Don't hesitate to ask for help from family members, friends, or professional caregivers.

Take Breaks: Schedule regular breaks to rest and recharge, even if it's just a few minutes throughout the day.

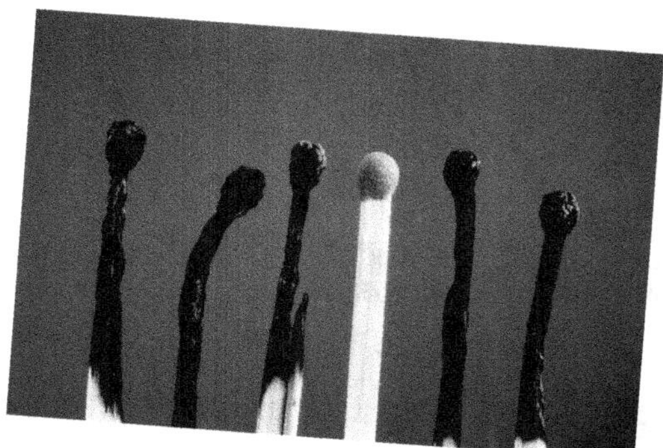

Strategies for Maintaining Your Own Mental and Physical Health

Maintaining your health is crucial to being an effective caregiver.

Physical Health:

Regular Exercise: Incorporate physical activity into your routine, whether it's a daily walk, yoga, or a fitness class. Exercise helps reduce stress and improve overall health.

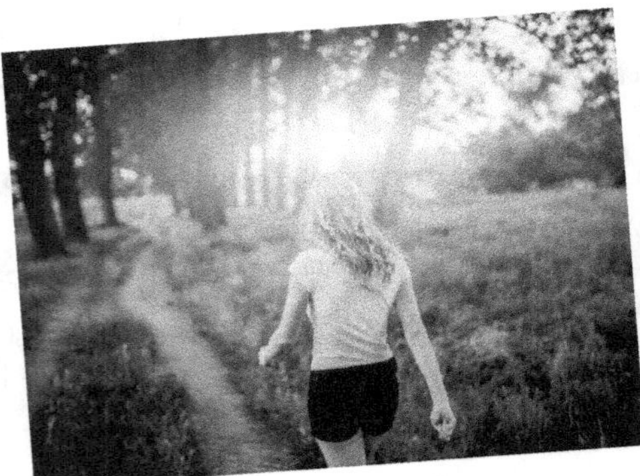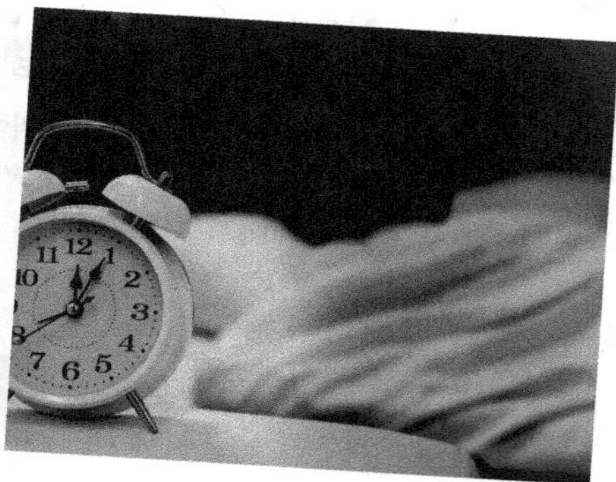

Balanced Diet: Eat a nutritious diet rich in fruits, vegetables, whole grains, and lean proteins. Avoid excessive caffeine and sugar.

Sleep Hygiene: Prioritize sleep by maintaining a regular sleep schedule, creating a comfortable sleep environment, and avoiding screens before bedtime.

Mental Health:

Mindfulness and Relaxation: Practice mindfulness, meditation, or deep-breathing exercises to reduce stress and promote mental clarity.

Hobbies and Interests: Engage in activities you enjoy to take your mind off caregiving duties and provide a sense of fulfilment.

Professional Help: Seek counselling or therapy if you're feeling persistently overwhelmed or depressed. Talking to a professional can provide valuable support and coping strategies.

Seeking Support from Fellow Carers and Professional Networks

Connecting with others who understand your experiences can provide invaluable support.

Support Groups: Join caregiver support groups, either in person or online, to share experiences, advice, and encouragement with others in similar situations.

Local Groups: Many communities offer support groups for caregivers, which can provide a sense of community and mutual support.

Online Communities: There are numerous online forums and social media groups where caregivers can connect, share stories, and offer support.

Workshops and Training: Attend workshops and training sessions to learn new skills and strategies for caregiving from trainers and coaches.

Balancing Caregiving Responsibilities with Personal Life

Balancing caregiving with your personal life is essential to avoid burnout and maintain your own well-being.

Set Boundaries: Establish clear boundaries between your caregiving duties and personal time. Communicate these boundaries with the person you're caring for and other family members.

Time Management: Use a calendar or planner to schedule caregiving tasks, personal activities, and breaks.

Say No: Learn to say no to additional responsibilities that can overwhelm you.

Personal Time: Make time for your hobbies, interests, and social activities.

Regular Activities: Schedule regular activities that you enjoy, such as reading, gardening, or meeting friends for coffee.

Social Connections: Maintain your social connections to avoid isolation. Spend time with friends and family who support and uplift you.

Respite Care: Utilize respite care services to take a break from caregiving duties.

Short-Term Relief: Respite care can provide short-term relief, whether it's for a few hours or a few days, allowing you to rest and recharge.

Long-Term Planning: Consider planning longer breaks, such as a weekend away, to fully disconnect and rejuvenate.

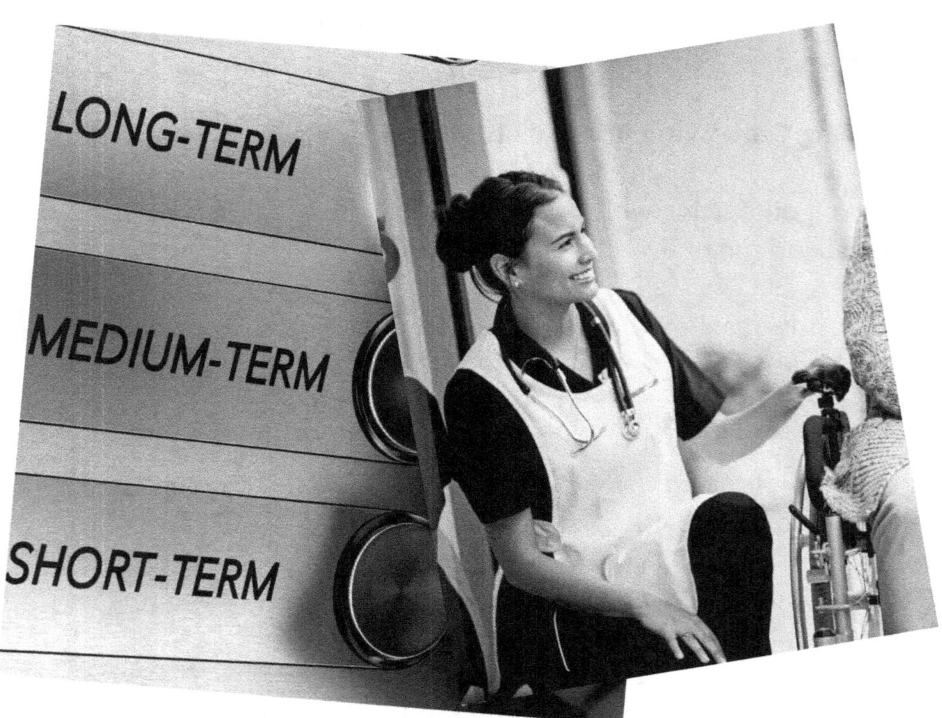

Conclusion

Self-care is not a luxury but a necessity for caregivers.

By recognizing and addressing caregiver burnout, maintaining your own mental and physical health, seeking support from fellow carers and professional networks, and balancing caregiving responsibilities with personal life, you can provide better care for your loved ones while ensuring your own well-being.

Prioritizing self-care allows you to be the best caregiver you can be, while also living a fulfilling and balanced life.

It's important that you keep the me in you.

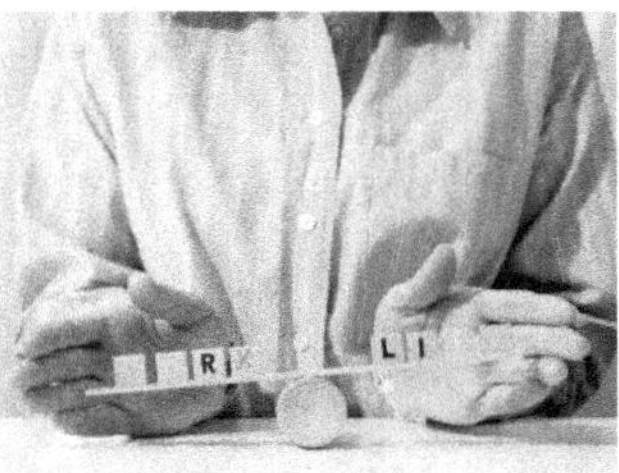

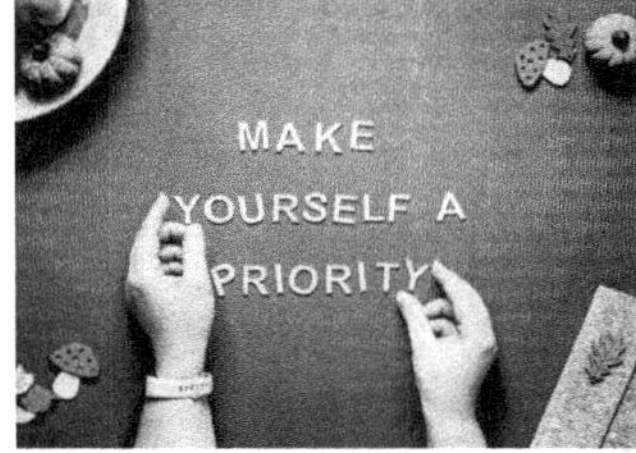

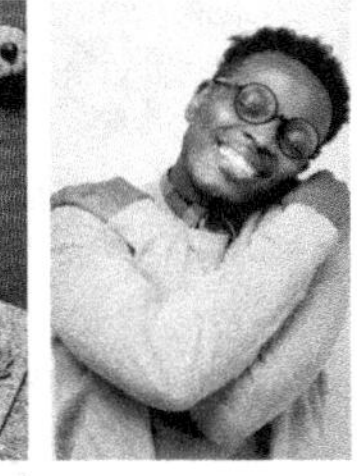

IMPROVES QUALITY OF LIFE

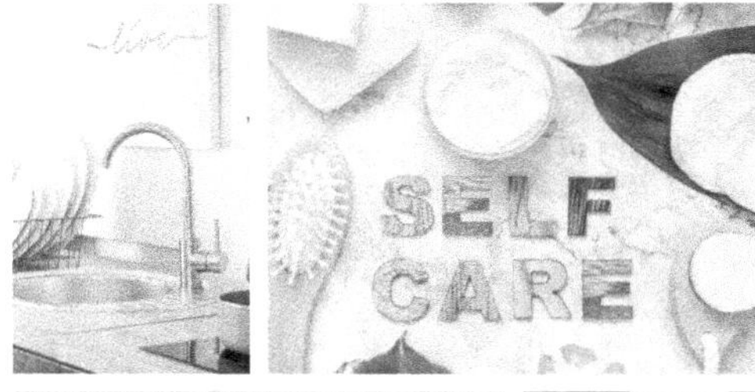

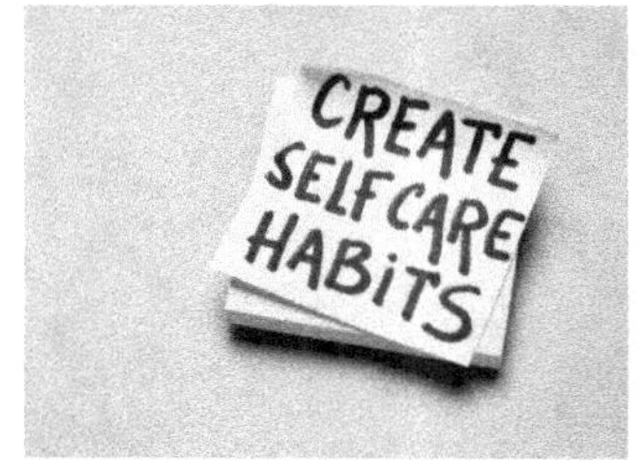

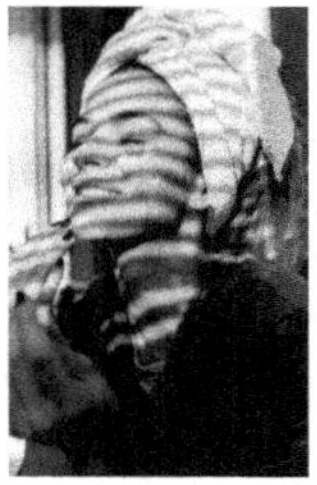

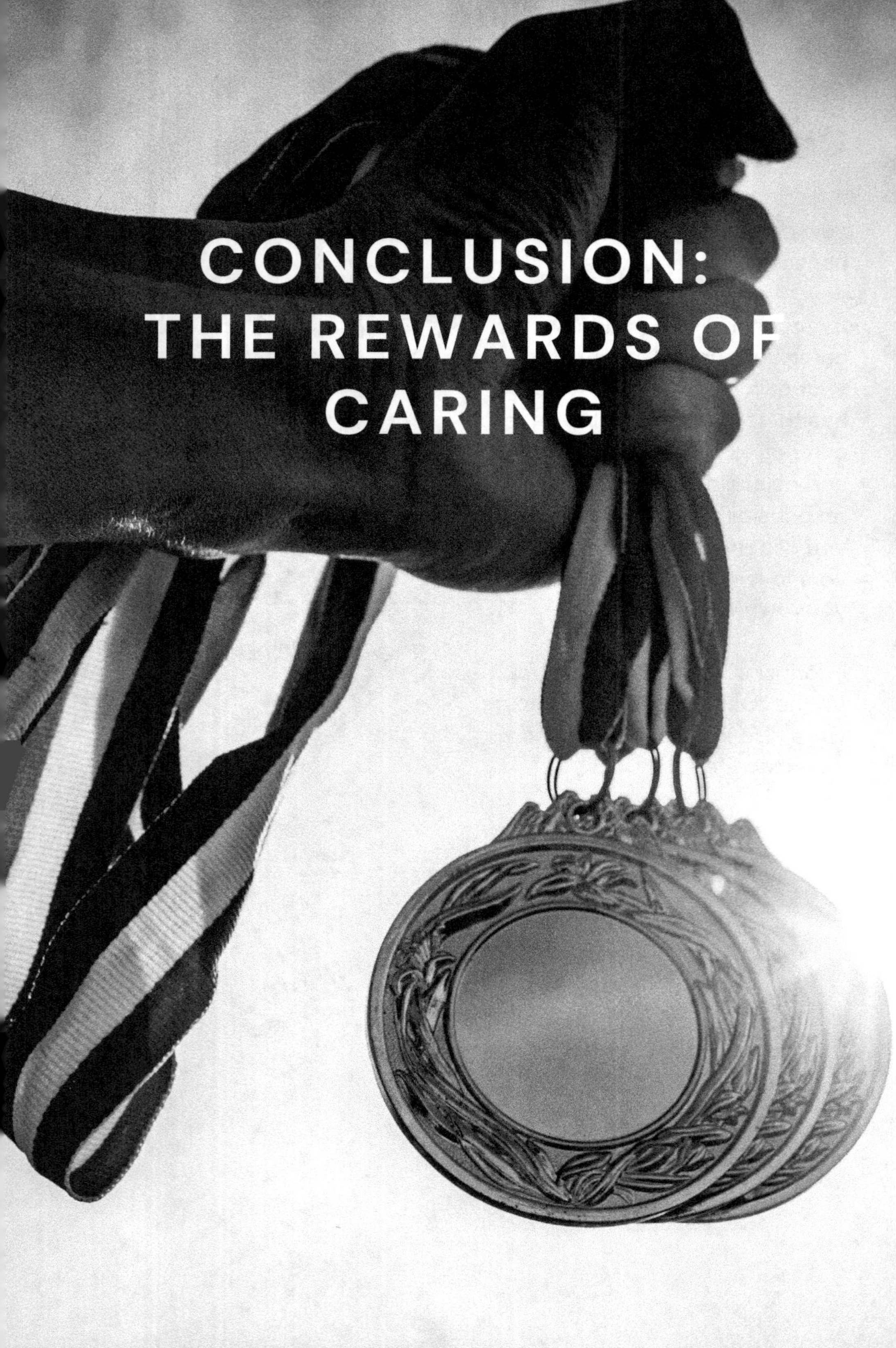

CONCLUSION:
THE REWARDS OF CARING

Reflecting on the Positive Impacts of Providing Care

Caring for someone, whether it's a family member or a non-relative, is a profound and impactful experience. Despite the challenges, the rewards of providing care are immense and deeply fulfilling.

This final chapter reflects on the positive impacts of caregiving, celebrates successes and milestones, and emphasizes the importance of continuing education and training for ongoing improvement.

Building Strong Bonds:

Caregiving often strengthens the relationship between the caregiver and the care recipient. Through shared experiences, mutual respect, and daily interactions, bonds are deepened and a sense

Personal Growth: The caregiving journey fosters personal growth and resilience. Caregivers often find themselves developing new skills, becoming more patient, compassionate, and understanding. The experience can lead to a profound sense of personal accomplishment and purpose.

Positive Outcomes: Witnessing the positive changes in the care recipient's health and well-being is incredibly rewarding. Whether it's improved physical health, increased emotional well-being, or enhanced quality of life, these outcomes validate the caregiver's efforts and dedication.

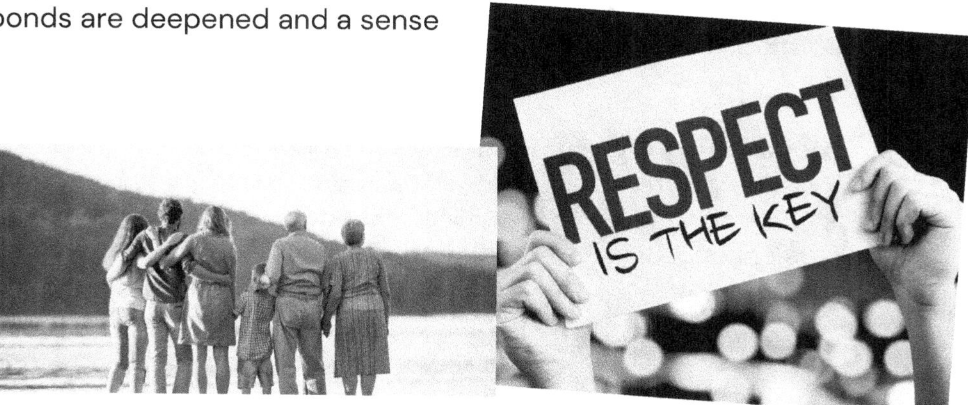

Celebrating Successes and Milestones in Caregiving

Acknowledging Achievements: Take time to acknowledge and celebrate the small and large achievements in caregiving. These might include successfully managing a difficult task, reaching a health milestone, or overcoming a significant challenge.

Milestone Moments: Celebrate milestone moments such as birthdays, anniversaries, and recovery milestones. These celebrations provide joy and create cherished memories for both the caregiver and the care recipient.

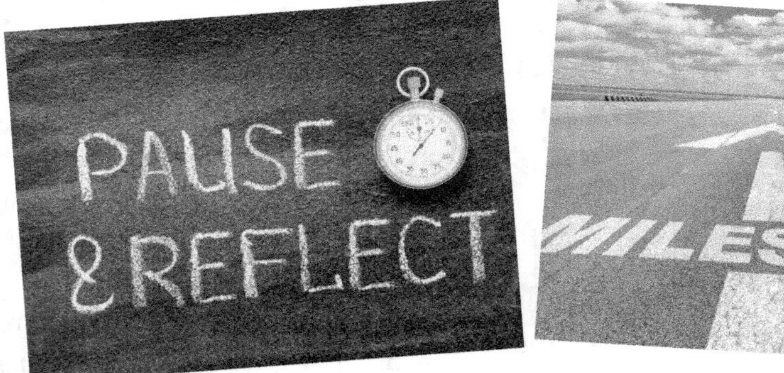

Reflective Practice: Regularly reflect on the caregiving journey. Keep a journal to document successes, challenges, and personal growth. Reflective practice helps caregivers recognize their progress and maintain a positive outlook.

Continuing Education and Training for Ongoing Improvement

Lifelong Learning: Caregiving is a dynamic and evolving field. Continuously seek out opportunities for education and training to stay informed about best practices, new techniques, and emerging research in caregiving.

Professional Development: Participate in workshops, webinars, and training sessions offered by experienced coaches and trainers. These professionals offer a wealth of advice and education, helping caregivers enhance their skills and knowledge.

Conclusion

The rewards of caregiving extend beyond the immediate tasks and challenges. It's about making a meaningful difference in someone's life, witnessing their growth and recovery, and knowing that your efforts contribute to their well-being and happiness. The fulfilment derived from caregiving is unparalleled, offering a deep sense of purpose and satisfaction.

As you reflect on your caregiving journey, celebrate the positive impacts and milestones you have achieved. Continue to seek out education and training opportunities to improve your skills and knowledge. Remember that professional coaches and trainers are invaluable resources, offering guidance, support, and expertise. Embrace the rewards of caring, knowing that your dedication and compassion make a profound difference in the lives of those you care for.

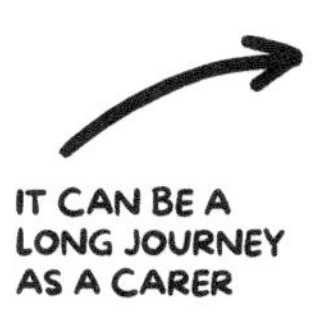

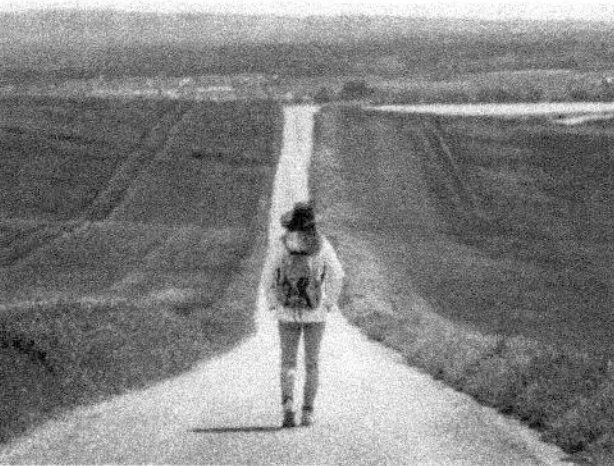

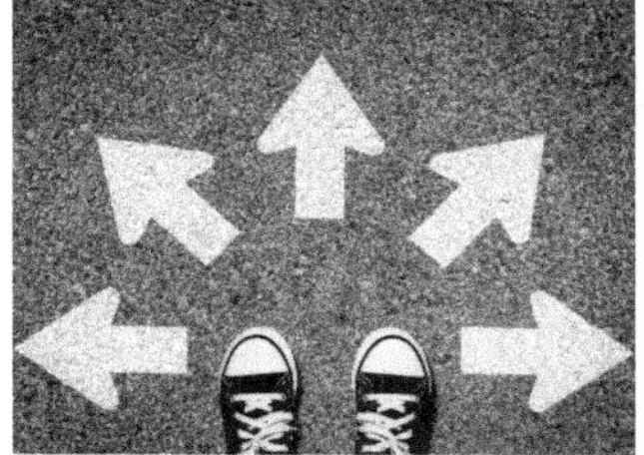

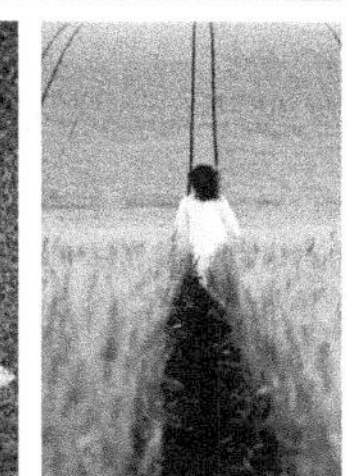

YOU WILL BE CHANGED FOR THE BETTER

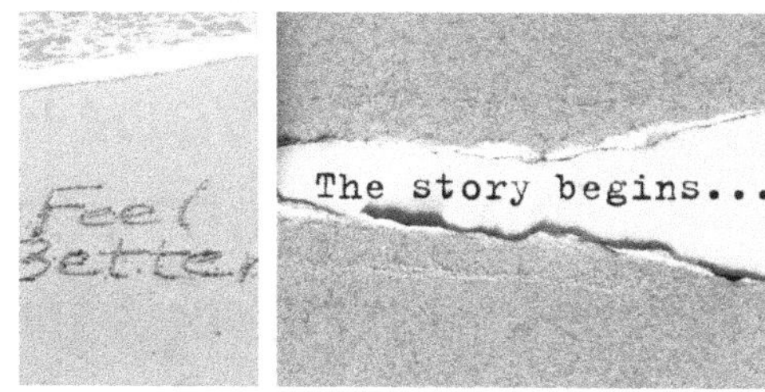

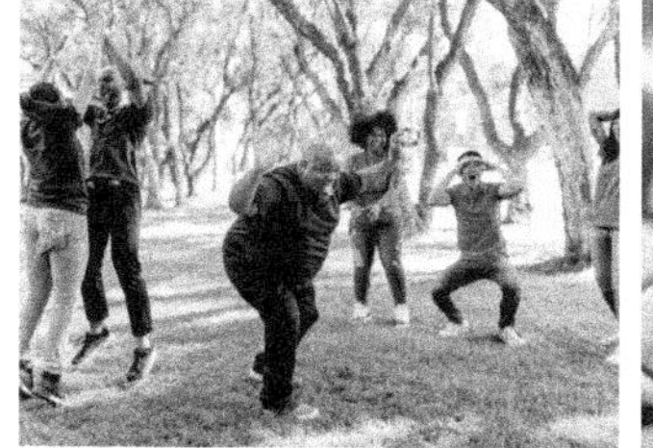

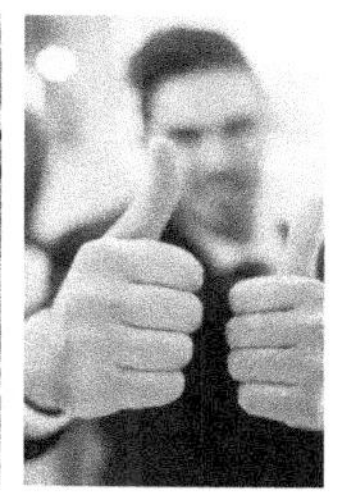

THE END

Here ends this book, but it could be the start of your journey. Keep looking forward but remember the past. Thankyou for reading!

ACKNOWLEDGEMENTS

I extend my heartfelt gratitude to all who have contributed to the creation of "I Can Be A Handful." Firstly, I wish to express my appreciation to the individuals whose stories have inspired this work. Your courage and resilience have illuminated the pages of this book, and I am deeply honored to have had the opportunity to share your experiences.

To the photographers whose captivating images adorn these pages, sourced from copyright-free platforms such as Canvas, thank you for your artistry and generosity. Additionally, I am grateful for the additional photographs captured by myself, Roy Langstaffe, which have enriched the visual narrative of this book.

Furthermore, I wish to acknowledge that any person mentioned in this book has had their names altered to safeguard their privacy and protect their identity.

Lastly, to my family, friends, and colleagues who have provided unwavering support and encouragement throughout this endeavor, I am profoundly grateful. Special mention to Angela, Jake, Charlie and Laurie. Your belief in me has been a constant source of strength, and I am indebted to each of you for your unwavering support.

With deepest appreciation,

A DIFFERENT KIND OF NORMAL

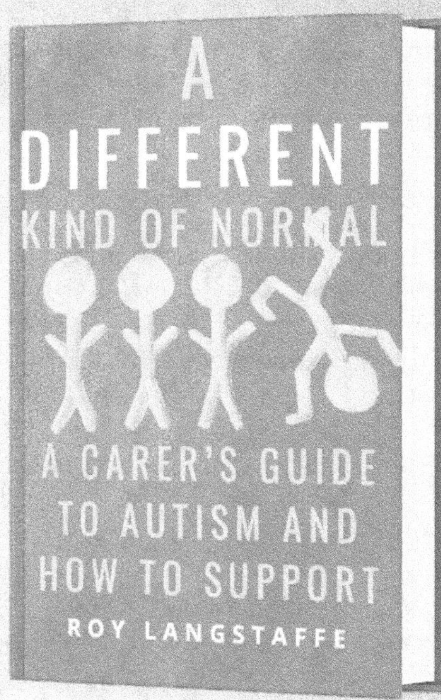

ROY LANGSTAFFE

A DIFFERENT KIND OF NORMAL: A CARER'S GUIDE TO AUTISM AND HOW TO SUPPORT IS ESSENTIAL FOR ALL CAREGIVERS, OFFERING PRACTICAL ADVICE, TIPS, AND INSPIRATION THROUGH INFORMATION AND REAL LIFE EXAMPLES OF HOW TO SUPPORT SOMEONE WITH AUTISM. IF YOU CARE, THIS IS ESSENTIAL READING!

DISCLAIMER